Biological Medicine
The Future of Natural Healing

Collected Papers
by

Dr. Thomas M. Rau, M.D.

Third, Extended Edition
December 2003

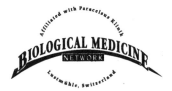

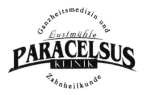

Biological Medicine Network
Verlag der Paracelsus Klinik Lustmühle

Third, Extended Paperback Edition, Dec. 2003

Published and distributed by

Verlag der Paracelsus Klinik Lustmühle
CH-9062 Lustmühle, Switzerland
Tel. ++41 (0)71 335 71 71
Fax ++41 (0)71 335 71 00
verlag@paracelsus.ch
www.paracelsus.ch

Distribution for USA & UK:
Biological Medicine Network
Marion Foundation
3, Barnabas Road
Marion
Massachusetts 02738-1421
USA
Tel. (508) 748 0816
Fax (508) 748 1976
bmn@marionfoundation.org
www.marionfoundation.org

Printed by

Kunz-Druck & Co. AG
CH-9053 Teufen, Switzerland

Biological Medicine – The Future of Natural Healing
ISBN 3-9522918-0-3

Dedication

To my grandmother "Omama"
who passed on to me her gift of intuitive knowing
about people and who is still with me in spirit

to my mother
who provided us with stability and a family life
and always believed in the good of humans

to my father
who imbued me with a spirit of independence
and taught me to follow my own thoughts

to my wife Elisabeth
who has supported my work through all these years
with dedication, patience and advice

and to my patients, from whom I have learned so much
about life, love, fear and values

Thomas Rau, 2003

Disclaimer

Although the author and publisher have exhaustively researched all sources to ensure the accuracy and completeness of the information contained in this book, we assume no responsibility for errors, inaccuracies, omissions or any inconsistency herein.

The information and procedures contained in this book are based on the professional experience at the Paracelsus Klinik. This book has been published for information and reference uses only. It is not intended in any respect as a substitute for a visit to a qualified doctor or other licensed health care practitioner. Every individual has a unique constitution and no method of treatment is useful for everyone. If you have a medical problem, please consult your qualified doctor or natural health care practitioner. The publishers and author are not responsible for any adverse effects or consequences resulting from the use of any suggestions, procedures, techniques, protocols, remedies or preparations discussed in this book.

Contents

Regulation Test Methods

About the Paracelsus Clinics

Acknowledgments

These papers on Biological Medicine were written in German over many years, both for our patients and for medical journals. The first edition of this book has been created due to the demand from many patients and through the initiative of Monica Bryant, who searched out and brought these papers together to help bring out more information on our Paracelsus approach to Biological Medicine. This third and widely extended edition was compiled due to the very positive response to the two former editions. It contends many more basic articles, but also descriptions on many more diagnoses and treatment schedules.

In looking back over how these papers came to be written and how my dedication to the English-speaking countries and patients grew, I would like to thank some "key-persons" in this development:
My dear teacher and now close friend Dr. Konrad Werthmann, who was the first to ask me to join him as teacher in his educational seminars. We have taught many seminars together over 12 years with the help of Mr. Reiner Kehlbeck, Director of Sanum-Kehlbeck in Germany. Chrystyne Jackson (Founder of Pleomorphic Products Sales Inc.), who brought me "over" to the U.S. as teacher. Chrystyne was my first supporter and organizer of seminars, when I was totally unknown to the U.S. Her support helped me very much and "rooted" me into the U.S.

For many years Mrs. Margie and Mr. Michael Baldwin, the Founders of The Marion Foundation, helped me by organizing all my seminars and spreading the word of Paracelsus all over the world. Not only that, but my friend Michael is also my business and strategic advisor in U.S. If, as a doctor, I hadn't had such a structuring, organizing and supportive person in the background, I would never be where I am today. We founded our "Biological Medicine Network" together, in the hope of creating a doctors network for Paracelsus' Biological Medicine to spread throughout the U.S., and to provide information about Biological Medicine for foreign patients. Out of this wonderful partnership grew a wider dimension of connections with very interesting people with spiritual and intellectual qualities, which become more and more important to me.

Mary and Al Shands, the owner of our affiliate Paracelsus Foxhollow Clinic in Crestwood KY, have also contributed to the important work of Biological Medicine by building up their most beautiful clinic, where Paracelsus Biological Medicine is practised in combination with Anthroposophical Medicine. Thank you, Mary and Al, for having such a trust in me and for letting me do all my work and seminars in your beautiful clinic!

Many friends supported me in the U.S., in seminars as teachers. But mainly – the U.S. and other foreign countries would never mean the same to me without these dear friends, who understand medicine in a similar way and who enabled a continuous communication and growth: James Odell, Soram Khalsa, Byron Braid, Dinos Xidas, Robert Zieve, Ahmed Al Shafei, Hennie Fitzpatrick, but also Dan Beilin and in the early years Scott Moyer, Dan Dunphy, David Nye, Harvey Bigelsen and some others!

Very important: all my work in foreign countries, all the endless time I spent in seminars and in our affiliate clinics was only possible because my partners and colleagues at home supported my work during all these years at the main Centre, the Paracelsus Klinik Lustmühle, Switzerland. Most of all I have to thank to my friend, Mr. Jürg Binz, President of the Paracelsus Klinik Lustmühle, my main partner in the Paracelsus Group, and my friend Dr. Victor von Toenges. Both have provided great stability and wisdom in the Paracelsus Klinik since our co-operation started and brought me to a deeper understanding of nature, human beings and medicine, but also clear determination and business strategies!

The first edition of this book was initially made possible through the hard work of Monica Bryant, Director of our Biological Medicine Network U.K. She compiled, supervised translations and edited the "pieces" to the first edition of this book! A really big effort – I would have never done it without her detail-oriented and conscientious work!

The significant extention to this third edition mainly was brought together by our "seminar officer" Mr. Ronald J. Sutter, who organized the total new compilation with all the details!

I owe you a special debt of thankfulness, Monica and Ronny.

Dr. Thomas M. Rau, M.D., December 2003

Note from the Editor

The Germanic European tradition of natural healing known as "Biological Medicine" is now attracting worldwide attention. However there is very little information available for patients and practitioners in English. So the Biological Medicine Network, a member of the Paracelsus group, operating in Switzerland, the U.S., the U.K. and Cyprus, is delighted to be able to publish a collection of papers and articles, written by Dr. Thomas M. Rau, M.D., co-founder and Medical Director of the Paracelsus Klinik Lustmühle.

Dr. Rau is a respected authority on this expanded form of naturopathic medicine, working together with his international team of doctors, dentists and other practitioners at the Paracelsus Clinics in Switzerland, the United States, and the cooperative clinic in Cyprus. Together they have developed a model of integrated medicine, which combines modern diagnostic and therapeutic equipment with a uniquely wide range of natural healing methods and remedies and holistic dentistry.

Presented in this book, is a compilation of papers written by Dr. Rau between 1993 and 2003. Bringing them together has inevitably resulted in some overlap of content and perhaps some inconsistencies. However, these articles are of real and lasting value for the understanding of the complex and integrative nature of Paracelsus Biological Medicine. They describe the general foundations and principles of Paracelsus Medicine and give many examples of specific applications.

There are various terms in this book which may be unfamiliar to the "orthodox" medical world. These are primarily from the work of Prof. Dr. Günther Enderlein, a German pioneer of pleomorphism. His work builds a central core of Paracelsus Biological Medicine. It describes the dynamic processes underlining diseases and their healing, but also the principles behind the phenomenal isopathic and immune biological remedies of the Sanum Kehlbeck company in Germany.

The theories of Enderlein and Homotoxicology are an integral part of Paracelsus Biological Medicin and we trust that readers will want to read further about these fundamental and dynamic views of health.

As the different articles were originally published in "Explore" or "Sanum-Post" or just used by the BMN, the spellings and even some terms may vary. The few papers that were translated by and published in "Explore – For the Professional" are reproduced in this book with the kind permission of Chrystine Jackson of Explore Publications in U.S.. They may perhaps show the prefix "Pleo" for Sanum products.

We also want to thank the Sanum company and the Semmelweiss Verlag for letting us use some of their translations of Dr. Rau's articles. And many thanks especially to Reiner Kehlbeck for his long term support in spreading the word of Dr. Rau in the "Sanum Post". These articles have a cooperative Copyright© for Dr. Rau and Semmelweiss Verlag.

The first, much smaller edition of this book came together in time for the first UK Biological Medicine lecture by Dr. Rau, held in London in October 2002. It was compiled at this time by Monica Bryant from BMN U.K. We want to thank her and her team again for the tremendous work she did, and also for showing us the need for making an extended edition for a larger readership.

Having been involved in this fields for over 15 years, we have always seen the healing potential of Biological Medicine, especially in chronic, autoimmune and infectious diseases. But we also have realized the vital importance of having information and education in English. Therefore the Paracelsus Klinik founded the Biological Medicine Network (BMN) to spread the knowledge of Paracelsus Biological Medicine in English speaking countries – and to publish further information for lay people and practitioners.

Our wish is that this book may contribute to open hearts and minds to the true importance of Paracelsus Biological Medicine.

Ulrich B. Schelling　　　　　　　Ronald J. Sutter
Co-Director of BMN　　　　　　　Publication Secretary
　　　　　　　　　　　　　　　　Paracelsus Clinics Switzerland

Switzerland and U.S., Dec. 2003

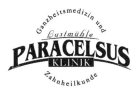

Introduction by Dr. Thomas Rau, M.D.

I have a deep commitment to Biological Medicine and have been privileged to witness many successful treatments over two decades in my practice at the Paracelsus Klinik. Integrated Biological Medicine is a profound approach to natural healing and can be very effective, especially when patients are committed to making the dietary and lifestyle changes that are also necessary. To understand our biological approach to health requires a different view of what the disease process is, compared to the currently held beliefs of conventional medicine.

To learn Biological Medicine as a whole, you need a completely different way of thinking. That is, thinking in terms of "regulation" and "information" and the idea that all diseases have their purposes. Seen in this light, symptoms are never diseases, but rather are signs of regulation. The human being is a part of nature and reacts like everything else in nature. So Biological Medicine is never about treating diseases, but is mainly about supporting the individuals in their particular reactions according to their differing constitutional types.

The biological doctor has to train his feeling for analogies (correspondences) in order to be able to understand the relationships between nature and a patient's symptoms. For me, this involved over ten years of attending courses following my medical training, studying with many alternative doctors, reading books, practising the new methods that I learned and listening to my patients. As ever, this process of learning always continues.

This holistic and biological approach to medicine is so completely different to conventional allopathic medical thinking that it will probably never be possible to teach it at medical schools or put it into repeatable treatment protocols. One can only be a biological doctor with a deep dedication to helping and healing, accepting that Biological Medicine is always the primary focus of care. It supports human reactions and never suppresses them, because these reactions always have their meaning, which we attempt to understand. In addition, being a biological doctor also means understanding that allopathic medicine is only complementary and secondary to Biological Medicine.

When Biological Medicine is subjected to the "scientific" methods commonplace today, with their statistical studies and double-blind trials, it will always fail. This gives the appearance that holistic treatments are not effective. On the contrary, we need to be proud of the fact that biological medicine often fails these studies, because the basic premise of these studies is wrong. They do not reflect the reality that the human being exists on a higher level than that which is statistically controllable with standardised studies. I believe that you can never standardise humans into one, or even several, variables. To really want to know about the effects of our treatments, I ask patients about their changes in attitude towards life, their understanding of their symptoms, and their intent to change themselves.

Trying to understand and study homeopathy allows you a very deep insight into the human character, its archetypal reactions, and the meaning and structure of personalities. This study takes you to a deeper level of information, into the very dimensions that make human beings the individuals that they are. Homeopathy therefore always has to be an important part of education for a holistic doctor, in part because the study of homeopathy also educates us about our own character. To truly learn Biological Medicine involves changing yourself, finding new interests and guidance in your life. It is believing in the good of nature, of which we and our patients are an integral part.

Isopathy and Enderleinian thinking is fundamental, because it teaches us that everything in humans is dynamic, always changing and reacting. It reminds us that we are most intensively part of the earth and nature, out of which we develop and live, and to which we return. Bacteria, viruses, and other microorganisms, which are commonly thought to be the causes of diseases, develop within us. These microbial forms exist within us as part of our cellular structure, normally in the form of proteins. The internal milieu that we create for ourselves through our diet and lifestyles changes these microorganisms, and by so doing, changes our predisposition to various diseases.

This book is intended to provide information about our Paracelsus Klinik approach to disease, regulation and Biological Medicine. The collection of papers is by no means a complete representation of my work today. However, they can be seen as some of the stepping stones in my own journey to understanding the essential keys to natural healing. Although my learning continues and my practice develops regularly to include new diagnostic and treatment methods, these papers still provide a foundation upon which my thinking and practice are built. I sincerely hope that you will find my papers of interest, not only to your understanding of Biological Medicine but also for your own well-being.

Dr. Thomas M. Rau, M.D.
December 2003

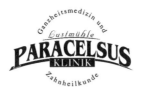

1

On the Nature of Biological Medicine

Introduction

At the Paracelsus Klinik Lustmühle and the ventures connected with it, a form of medicine is practised which we call "Integrated Biological Medicine". It is based on knowledge of orthodox medicine, physiology and biochemistry, but integrates various ancient forms of traditional natural healing, which have been tried and tested for thousands of years. On the other hand it also follows the very latest findings of scientific theory, physics and biochemistry.

The patient is regarded as a whole being, we never consider only the diseased organ. We never treat the symptoms themselves but the obstructed functions and causes, which can lead to the appearance of the symptoms. This paper offers a brief description of a few of the fundamental approaches that we use in Biological Medicine.

The Paracelsus Klinik is the first and only clinic in Switzerland where, over a period of more than ten years, all the methods described below have been used consistently and in a wide range of combinations by doctors and dentists.

Integrated Biological Medicine is particularly well suited to the treatment of chronic and nebulous diseases. It is basic therapy that can be used as the primary form of treatment in all types of illness. Therefore it is incorrect to call it "complementary medicine" as it is used not merely as a supplement to orthodox medicine but as a form of treatment in its own right.

Integrated Biological Medicine integrates the knowledge from different natural healing systems and philosophical teachings into a form of medical treatment that approaches the patient as a whole, taking into consideration their dynamic processes. The doctor or therapist who practises Integrated Biological Medicine needs basic knowledge of physiology and human biochemistry, as these theories best explain the basic metabolism and cell reactions of human beings. For this reason, a previous study of science is also of advantage.

Integrated Biological Medicine, as practised intensively for more than ten years at the Paracelsus Klinik Lustmühle, integrates Chinese meridian theory, Ayurvedic and European Paracelsian theory of constitution, phytotherapy, homeopathy, and also traditional humoral therapies such as detoxification, stimulation therapy of a physical type and hydrotherapy. Homotoxicology is an important component of Biological Medicine. But one very important element which supplements the conventional natural healing processes, is **strict milieu theory.** Everything in human beings which "flows", every movement of material and dynamic adjustment to a steady state condition is dependent on the **mesenchymal milieu,** i.e. the acid-base situation, the protein situation and the **orthomolecular conditions** in the inner compartments.

The mesenchymal (= interstitial) system works through all the tissues and links all the organs with one another. The mesenchyme is the specific carrier of all information and the instinctive (involuntary) function systems. Many diseases, in particular chronic diseases and disorders, are caused by an obstruction to the flow of information and the metabolism of the mesenchyme. Molecules and clusters (conglomerates of molecules) of water are important as the only carriers of information in the body, but directed polysaccharide molecules in the ground substance also act as other types of information carriers. This fact also partially explains the phenomenon of homeopathy, as it seems probable that the "information" from homeopathic remedies can modify the characteristics of the clusters of water molecules.

Another approach, difficult to understand by way of modern medical teaching, is **pleomorphism** as defined by Professor Enderlein: its isopathic approach and milieu therapy are important for Biological Medicine. Bacteria and their antecedents, proteins, affect every system in humans and are vitally important to us – not only in the digestive system but also for cell metabolism (uptake of oxygen / coagulation) and the immune system (the bowel ensures the efficiency our immune system – see below). Therefore, according to the pleomorphistic theory, infectious diseases are not caused by bacteria, viruses or fungi; instead these pathogenic organisms can develop by pathological means into pathogens as the milieu changes.

Modern Integrated Biological Medicine is characterised by an enormous store of knowledge from the traditional medicine of China and India, and also the teachings in central Europe of Paracelsus von Hohenheim. On the other hand it also integrates the latest physical and biochemical discoveries regarding trace elements, free radicals, vitamins, amino acids – that is, orthomolecular and physical discoveries regarding the significance of membrane potential, redox potential, the benefits of oxygen, etc.

It seems important to us, however, that our medicine is characterised by this very enormity of experience. Experience of tradition by millions of people and over centuries from our point of view counts for more than supposedly "double–blind", "scientific" studies which are often nothing but reductionist ways of looking at things. Studies in which only single variables are compared and recorded in the human system – which, however, regularly contains within itself thousands of variables and dynamic alterations! It seems to us downright arrogant not to recognise traditional methods of healing because of their "unscientific" basis, although they are based on evidence and have been tried and tested over generations. But they are not recognised because their multifariousness does not allow them to be included in the non-dynamic and simplistic criteria of the conditions required for the study.

The concept of "regulation"

Biological Medicine speaks of **regulation** as a concept for the fine-tuning of the inner milieu and attaches great importance to this regulation. The ability to regulate is a precondition for the maintenance of an inner balance, even in a changing environment. Regulation is for the most part provided for by receptors in the **autonomic nervous system and limbic system,** by the mesenchyme, and also by the bowel, which is the largest organ in our bodies. But particularly the intact intestinal flora (our largest "organ" in terms of numbers of cells) and the **Peyer's lymph patches**

which are found in the submucous membrane (and which form 80 % of our lymphatic system) are what enable regulation and demarcation from the environment and have an important influence on the detoxification of the human body.

The bowel, the lymphatic system and the intestinal flora are therefore included in practically every course of integrated biological therapy. The bowel and its bacteria ensure the link to Mother Earth and are a deciding force in determining our parasympathetic nervous system's and our **ability to build ourselves up**. (See also the paper: The Intestine, Nutrition and Health)

The understanding that human beings are a part of the whole, i.e. of the earth and of creation, and are very closely connected to the earth for the whole of their life as well as before and after, colours the thinking behind holistic medicine most deeply in the manner of the anthroposophists and Paracelsus.

One further point has a different relative importance in Integrated Biological Medicine compared to the rather more statically aligned and organ-oriented theories of orthodox medicine:

The dynamics of all vital processes
All processes in the living organism are dynamic and all the organs are continually being destroyed and rebuilt. Every organ, even a diseased one, rebuilds itself, with a different rhythm for each organ. The lymphatic system, for example, has a regenerative dynamic of about three weeks, intestinal bacteria take a few days, and slowly regenerating tissues such as cartilage and bone take years. In this way every disease of an organ has a rhythm that must be taken into consideration during treatment. The treatment of a diseased organ in order to build it up must always be continued for as long as it takes for one or more regeneration cycles of the corresponding tissue to be completed.

But it is important to note that every organ renews itself, even a diseased one! When the milieu situation and the conditions for the build-up of new tissue are supported, then the newly forming tissue can develop better and become more resistant! This theory is of the greatest importance, as even in degenerative diseases of the organs (e.g. hepatitis, cartilage defects, osteoporosis, arteriosclerosis, etc) work must be done primarily on the conditions for building up the corresponding organ and on the "anabolic" ability of the body to build itself up. This is provided for by general milieu therapy, isopathy and orthomolecular "cell therapies".

Traditional Chinese medicine takes particular account of rhythmic renewal processes. Its **"five element theory"** explains the connections and rhythmic support of the different organs, one to another. It also explains the "energetic" and meridian connections between the different organs. Therefore Integrated Biological Medicine integrates the theories behind Chinese medicine in its approach.

Integrated Biological Medicine is therefore not simply a form of treatment with natural remedies instead of chemical medication, but a bringing back of the patient to a dynamic connection with the regulation processes and thus the laws and rhythms of Nature and the Earth.

However theoretical this sounds, the consistent implementation of it is logical and straightforward. Biological Medicine is simple, deals with living things and is straightforwardly logical – that is why it is bio-logical!

PARADIGMS OF BIOLOGICAL MEDICINE

In order to make it easier to understand, here are a few short explanations of the basic approaches of Biological Medicine:

1. Human beings become ill because of toxic overload.
The significance of heavy metals / organic toxins / dysbiotic toxins / fungal toxins
The **concept of toxic regulation blockades** is of the greatest importance in Biological Medicine. Influences that obstruct the delicate adjustments of the metabolism are the most important causes of disease. Natural healing experiences show that nowadays the **influence of toxins is the most important blockade to regulation**. In the forefront are the toxins from heavy metals (mercury, lead, palladium), other toxic metals (aluminium and nickel) but also organic toxins (e.g. preservatives in

foodstuffs, which however also "preserve" the vital processes as a result of their long-term accumulation).

Also of great significance are **microbial toxins**, e.g. from dental foci, chronic dysbiosis and/or fungal infestation. Toxins block normal regulatory and adaptation processes in the body by misdirecting metabolic processes, disrupt the behaviour of bacteria and compete with other, natural detoxification processes. Many toxic blocks to regulation can be simply proved by chemistry or fine energy, but unfortunately they are mainly disregarded in medical explanations.

Typical diseases which are frequently caused by toxins are ulcerative colitis, tumour diseases (combined with other factors), chronic fatigue syndrome, neuralgic pain (mostly combined with dental foci or chronic viral overload), multiple sclerosis, almost all allergies (mostly in combination with significant lack of trace elements), infections, etc.

Therefore in biological regulation medicine we always look for blockades to regulation, and for these particular regulation diagnostic methods are used.

The "barrel of disease"

Symptoms (in the illustration the over-flow from the barrel) first occur when the ability of the body to compensate (filling the barrel until it over-flows) is exhausted. This explains why just a few problems do not lead to symptoms or disease and can often be compensated for years on end. The method in Biological Medicine is such that where there are diseases and symptoms it is always possible to look for the reason why the "barrel" is filling: Toxic overloads / excess of acid / disturbance fields / weakness of the constitution / electromagnetic overloads and endobiontic overloads (see following).

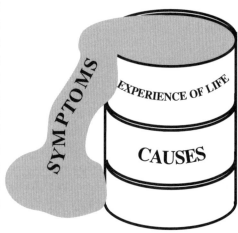

The main regulation blockades

- Foci, disturbance fields (e.g. teeth, old scars, old foci of infection)

- Chronic organic and inorganic toxic overloads

- Heavy metals from the teeth / preservatives / disinfectants

- Bacterial and fungal toxins

- Excess of acid / excess of protein in the mesenchyme / "building up of morbid matter"

- The build-up of free radicals (e.g. toxins or morbid matter from the normal cell metabolism which are not excreted)

- Chemotherapy products, antiphlogistics, etc., accumulated over a long period

- Food intolerances resulting in damage to the intestinal mucous membrane

- Long-term physical stress with overload of the sympathetic nervous system

2 Disease is the expression of a reduction in the body's ability to regulate itself and
the result of degenerative development.

The significance of Dr. Reckeweg's teachings / Homotoxicology, the onset of degeneration as the expression of the body's reduced ability to excrete and react.

Dr. H. H. Reckeweg, M.D., himself a great homeopath, initiated crucial developments in homeopathic science. His **six-phase teachings** explain the theory of Biological Medicine behind many issues: A healthy body can detoxify itself by normal excretion stools, urine, perspiration, etc. When the inner level of toxicity is raised, the body should recognise this and through self-regulation develop excretion symptoms such as vomiting, diarrhoea, increased sweating, high temperature, etc. But if it is suppressed or too lethargic, it develops instead a leucocytolitic form of "inner excretion": that is, an inflammatory and/or hyperergic reaction. If this too is suppressed (by medication or regulation blockades), the body stores up the toxins, which then cause deposition problems (like liver disorders, vascular disorders, circulatory problems, hypertonia, a high cholesterol level, etc., myoma, myogelosis, etc, etc). (= **Deposition Phase**). With long-term therapy, the deposition phase can mainly be made to regress.

According to the type of toxic overload, the toxins can enter the cells: the body even impregnates its own cells with toxins (free radicals), which can lead to changes in function of the cells. Examples of this are: thyroid problems, diabetes, heart failure, hormone disorders, etc. (= **Impregnation Phase**)

Long-term cell intoxifications can lead to irreversible damage to the cells and to tissue degeneration or tumours. Thus the doctor of Biological Medicine also regards cancers as a "degenerative development" (= **Degeneration or tumour phases**). Some typical degeneration phases are diseases of old age, lack of brainpower, arthosis, osteoporosis, cirrhosis, all problems of insufficiency. But frequently people who are still too young are affected by degenerative problems, which are then almost always the expression of influences restricting the body's regulatory mechanism.

Here too, in therapeutic terms, one can draw out a simple and logical consequence: problems of chronic degeneration or even tumour problems can be cured by inducing the body to increase cellular activity (with catalysts, trace elements, vitamins, etc.) and then supporting the body's ability to become inflamed and to excrete endotoxins.

Here biological regulation medicine is at odds with conventional "modern" medicine, which treats symptoms by suppressing them and inhibiting inflammation. In Biological Medicine we try to detoxify the cells, the mesenchyme and thus the whole body. On the other hand, the patient's powers of regeneration are built up, which in turn favours natural modification and the dynamics of the tissue.

Biological Medicine requires subtle **research methods** which show the doctor the state of reaction and the level of blockades in the patient:

Research methods in biological regulation medicine:

- Clinical examination of the patient

- Orthopantomography of the teeth and measurement of galvanic currents in the mouth

- Thermoregulation diagnosis

- Darkfield microscopic examination of the vital blood

- Holographic viewing of the blood crystallisation (dried layer test)

- Investigation for toxic chemicals, testing for heavy metals and hair analysis

- Testing of the autonomous nervous system using rhythmic procedures (including Heart Rate Variability)

- Measurement of redox potential and the acid-base milieu in lymph, urine and blood

- Electroacupuncture for the measurement of the "energy flow" in the mesenchyme

- Fine regulatory tests from traditional medicine such as kinesiology, radiesthesia

These regulation testing methods do not only show how regulation is disturbed but also the disturbance foci, toxic overloads and even subtle information.

3. Disturbance foci trigger chronic diseases or make them worse

A disturbance focus is an underlying focus of inflammation which is not noticeable at the point of the focus but which can cause a remote interference via the mesenchyme or via the meridian system, the result being incorrect reactions in the remote organ. Disturbance foci are very frequently one of the joint causes of chronic diseases.

The disturbance foci which occur most frequently (approximately 80%) are:

- Dead (root-treated) teeth

- Old scars or chronic inflammation of the tonsils or nasal sinuses

- Chronic mis-colonisation of the bowel with underlying irritation of the intestinal crypts

In chronic illnesses which do not heal using other natural healing methods, one should always consider disturbance foci. Frequently we see disturbance foci as the cause of MS, polyarthritis, back pain, headache and neuralgia. Only subtle regulation testing can show the presence of disturbance foci, such as electroacupuncture, milieu tests and thermoregulation diagnosis according to Professor Rost. Disturbance foci cannot be discovered using normal blood tests.

THE DISTURBANCE FOCUS

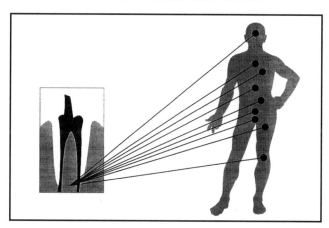

The disturbance focus
(= Underlying inflammation which can only be sensed by it remote effect)

- Needs a "trigger", that is, a second cause

- Can remain silent for years!

4. All diseases are multi-causal and depend on the constitution of the patient.

The constitution, not the diagnosis, is important – Homeopathy / constitution theory / five element theory.

Very many diseases are "idiopathic", i.e. their cause is not known. But only because they always have different causes which can be combined quite individually in different patients, depending on the **patient's constitution.**

A wide-ranging search for different causes is therefore very important in chronic diseases, and so is identification of the patient's constitution. Every type of constitution is sensitive to different forms of stress, as we can see in homeopathy with its highly polished teachings on the constitution.

It is exactly in this sort of disease that as many contributory causes as possible must be found – like the little stones of a mosaic, they only create a picture when they are all put together, for example, the **"Allergy Temple"**. A good example of this is allergies or asthma. The allergen is usually only a triggering factor. But the root of the problem is caused by

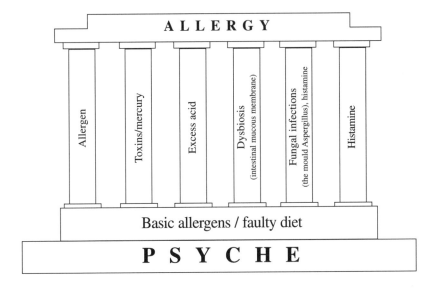

milieu factors and contamination which alter the immune system's capabilities: food allergies, heavy metal contamination, dysbioses or fungi, lack of trace elements. Thus people with allergies can be healed without the possible of eliminating the allergen, but on an individual basis and only by removing the contributory causes.

Theory of constitutions is of the greatest importance for Biological Medicine and can be found again and again in practically all the tried and tested traditional methods of healing, although under different names. Only "modern" orthodox western medicine pushes the significance of the typically individual reactions by different patients into the background and treats diagnoses in a reproducible and non-individualised manner. This, of course, has the big advantage that orthodox medicine can be learnt in "cookbook fashion" and can also be reproduced by everybody. But it has the disadvantage that medicine is not performed for the benefit of the person but "against a diagnosis" and loses its artistic character.

In the following section I shall list a few different descriptions of constitutions, which come from the teachings from different healing traditions:

Traditional Chinese medicine

- **Meridian constitution types** (according to Dr. Rau, **"Function circle types"**)   Liver-Gall Bladder – Heart-Small Intestine – Stomach-Spleen/Pancreas – Lung-Large intestine – Kidney-Bladder

- *The 5-element cyclic phases and their characters:* Wood (spring) – Fire (summer) – Earth (late summer) – Metal (autumn) – Water (winter)

Ayurvedic medicine

Kapha, Pitta and Vatta types

These three types correspond astoundingly to the constitutional types in Kretschmer's teachings and Enderlein's three main types: congestion, inflammation and degeneration types equivalent to the Mucor, Penicillium and Aspergillus constitutions

Enderleinian isopathic constitution types

Mucor, Penicillium and Apergillus types

Prof. Dr. Günther Enderlein, the founder of isopathy and developer of the theory of pleomorphism, observed that when an endobiontic high valency prevails, there is normally is an associated inclination to a specific group of diseases, as well as a typical type of constitution and character of the patient.

- **The Mucor type** inclines to congestion, in many aspects corresponds to the syphilitic type, tends towards diseases of the body fluids, of the vascular and circulation system and, problems with the metabolism and glandular system. In many ways this type is also like Kretschmer's leptosome-entodermal type.

- **The Penicillium type** inclines to infectious diseases, reactions of the excess type, ulcerations, inflammations of the bacterial kind, possibly with cell reorganisation. In many ways this type is similar to the sycotic miasm.

- **The Aspergillus type** is the psoric type who in youth tends towards allergies and lymphatic problems. However, as this type grows older, degenerative and chronic problems begin to appear. This type's predispositions include diseases of the connective tissue, the legs and spine, the brain and the kidneys. The basic disease is tuberculosis or in the homeopathic sense the "tuberculinic" reaction.

Kretschmer's theory of constitution

- **Leptosome-ectodermal-arthenic** (schizothymic-introverted)

- **Normosome-athletic-mesodermal**

- **Pyknic-entodermal** (cyclothymic-depressive-extroverted)

Hahnemann's theory of miasms

As well as describing the constitutional dispositions of the main homeopathic polychrests (i.e. of the individual important remedies) Hahnemann, the great founder of homeopathy, also created a reaction typology which distinguishes between three principal reaction types; these almost exactly correspond to the main Enderleinian types and for that reason attract again and again the same constitutional remedies but also feature specific reaction types and as a result specific types of disease. When he described the accompanying constitutional types, Hahnemann took as his starting point the typical diseases of his time:

- **The syphilitic constitution**
  A syphilitic person tends towards destructive reactions: diseases of the metabolism, congestive and irritable diseases, diseases of the legs and spine, as well as in his/her behavioural tendency towards fiery-impulsive, erratic but also destructive reactions.

- **The sycotic constitution**
  Stems from sycosis (= disease of the condylomata, gonorrhoea): an intermediate type, but with tendency towards overflowing reactions, infectious diseases, in effect the penicillium type.

- **The psoric constitution**
  From psora, which stands for 'scabies', common at that time, a degenerative type of skin disease. The psoric person reacts too little, tends towards atopical reactions, degenerative diseases and neuro-degenerative diseases. However, their character is predictable and clear, though often also rigid, systematic and "dry", orderly.

Carl Hutter's theory of types (naturals)

Carl Hutter is the founder of pathophysiognomy, the theory of postural expression and a person's appearance. Hutter has described an enormous number of links between posture, bodily build, the physiognomy of the face and people's character. He too describes three main types, which he calls "naturals".

- **The resting and eating natural**
  A person with a sturdy body and stomach, calm, practically inclined, simple, the lymphatic type.

- **The moving and doing natural**
  Inclined to be energetic and masterful, quick to perceive and react, large, dynamic, a muscular person, and a person who moves a lot.

- **The thinking and feeling natural**
  A person with fine features and large forehead, a strong spiritual/psychic radiance. An introverted thinker, musician type.

The important thing about recognising the patient's constitution is that one can treat in a much more individual manner or also recognise what will be their physical reactions to treatment. But it also enables you to advise the patient on preventive measures and to recognise disease tendencies. According to their basic constitution, the patient will also encounter a specific type of problems and themes in their life, time and time again. Constitutions therefore also have a strong influence on the patient's psychology and how he or she experiences life. This understanding is what also the **homeopathic theory of constitution** works with: the assignment of a very specific experience, disease tendency and clinical picture to the individual homeopathic remedies.

5. Nutrition is an important factor in healing
Or – the power for the organism to be renewed comes from Nature's ability to re-build (anthroposophic theory) and is supported by diet!

The intestine is our largest organ by far and contains as many bacteria as there are cells in the human body. The intestinal mucous membrane is the organ, which can replace and re-build itself the fastest. Both these powers of renewal and the intestinal bacteria affect our whole being and are to a great extent dependent on what we eat. A person's ability for recovery and restoration – especially if someone has a degenerative illness – must therefore in turn be a building-up process of the colon. That is why individual changes in diet are of the greatest importance in chronic diseases. Food should be wholesome, if possible in its natural state and very low in animal protein, preferably vegetarian and with no cows' milk.

Food intolerances are extremely common and are commonly the cause of chronic diseases, where often the connection with food has not been made: practically all allergies, skin complaints, rheumatism (especially polyarthritis), behavioural problems in children, practically all infections, etc.

In the long term a healthy diet is the most important factor in the treatment of chronic resistance to health. (For further thoughts on this subject see the paper – The Intestine, Nutrition and Health)

6. The intestine connects us to the Earth

It connects us to the Earth through the intestinal bacteria and through the fact that our food provides us with everything essential for renewal and what we need as building materials in our body. The bacteria make sure that all this works and also detoxify us. They also "pre-digest" many materials – live in wonderful symbiosis with human beings: they are actually part of us. They ensure that our immune system functions by continually stimulating it. They come from the earth, and they are also what return us to the earth after our death. They give us anabolic and ethereal powers to shape and build ourselves up.

The care of the intestinal flora by means of isopathic therapy and fibre-rich vegetarian food is of the greatest importance. But it frequently happens that the patient requires a specific course of therapy over a longer period of time with trace elements (e.g. molybdenum), vitamins and amino acids, as well as adjustment of the acid-base balance, so that their intestinal flora can once again develop properly. Enemas, colonic irrigation and specific bacterial remedies can speed up this process considerably. The practical significance of these associations is striking: diseases caused by the intestine are a frequent occurrence: migraines, allergies, lung complaints of various types, back problems in the lumbar region, epigastric flatulence, nausea, chronic constipation and excess weight!.

Here too Biological Medicine has a few subtle testing methods which show whether the intestinal flora are intact: thermoregulation diagnosis, comprehensive testing of stools for the ability to digest and absorb, as well as darkfield microscopy, which demonstrates the dynamic processes of the development of bacteria on blood or other testing media.

The special point about Integrated Biological Medicine is, therefore, that it combines individual, different methods of natural healing and links modern orthomolecular knowledge with the constitutional type of the patient. During therapy the disease of the organ remains in the background in contrast to the re-attainment of the dynamic regulative condition of the whole patient.

A summary of Dr. Rau's lecture on "New ways in Medicine" at the Medical Congress at Glarus, 20 – 22 September 2001.

Dr. Thomas Rau, M.D.
Paracelsus Klinik Lustmühle,
9062 Lustmühle (bei St.Gallen)
Switzerland

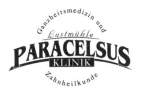

2.

The Clinical Picture of Hyperproteinemia and Hyperacidity

Introduction

Every biological therapy and every isopathic therapy (Sanum therapy) is exclusively oriented to the organism's regulatory system. It influences the organism's adaptability and its internal milieu – and thus the reactions or regulatory processes in the organism. Thus, the biological therapist views each symptom as the expression of a specific regulatory effort on the part of the organism and uses it as a guide to determine which metabolic processes are active, which are disturbed or in need of assistance. Therefore, he never treats the symptom itself, but supports the system's goals instead. For example, inflammation and its accompanying pain is not an ailment per se; it is, instead, the expression of the organism's efforts to digest or phagocytose toxins or defective proteins by means of inflammation. The therapist lends support to the goals of the inflammation by stimulating leukocytic systems and assists circulatory conditions or strengthens the lymphatic system in its diversionary capacity. This way, painful turgor can be reduced and the goals of the inflammation supported. But if – as in the present example – inflammatory processes are suppressed by anti-inflammatories, then the body cannot attain its goal, which is processing toxins, and tissue becomes burdened with toxins, proteins or immune complexes. It will in the future be more susceptible to recurring tissue disturbances.

Therefore, the biological therapist attempts to improve the adaptability and responsiveness of the organism by working at the regulatory system level.

In their work, Pischinger, Sander and Wendt have written that the **integrity of the interstitial system** is the most important prerequisite for good tissue regulation and responsiveness, since all the fine material data (but also cellular material exchange) takes place in these minuscule interstitial spaces. The conductivity and transportability of the interstitial fluid depends on the:

- Protein content of the interstitium

- Acid-base balance (pH value)

- Mineral and trace element content

- Endobiontic infestation, particularly the endobiontic high valences, which is a consequence of the first three criteria

Hence, it is crucial that every biological therapy be preceded by a normalization (adjustment) of the interstitial milieu. In other words: it has been shown that every chronically ill person exhibits a dislocation of the inner milieu (the condition of the interstitium). This explains why biological therapy can never be symptom-oriented but must always orient itself to the interstitium.

THE SIGNIFICANCE OF
DARKFIELD MICROSCOPY
IN CLINICAL PRACTICE

- Milieu ?
- Excess protein ?
- Immune system activity
  - -> Protits ?
  - -> Leukocyte mobility ?
- Endobiont infestation ?
- Cell resistance ? / Cellular respiration ?

- Primary Starting Point for therapy:
  - -> Diversion ?
  - -> Deproteinization ?
  - -> Endobiont treatment ?
  - -> Immune system stimulation

This means that Sanum therapy cannot be applied with respect to indications lists only, but must absolutely be administered on an individual basis. Enderlein describes this in his writings and points out that all isopathic therapy deals primarily with the milieu and that any development upward or downward of the endobiontic valences can only be achieved by a change in the milieu.

Any isopathic or immunobiological therapy must be accompanied by: treatment of the interstitial protein content with medications and dietetic measures; regulation of the acid-base balance; and – increasingly important these days – adjusting the trace element level. The fact that homeopathic and isopathic agents work better when administered along with trace elements had been noted even before Enderlein by Hahnemann in his later works, as well as by Rudolf Steiner. Our experience has very much confirmed this, as we have seen that isopathic agents combined with orthomolecular medicine or homeopathic trace elements (Sanum) work considerably better.

The issue of protein loading and the interstitial pH value will be dealt with thoroughly in the following section.

The evaluation of tissue pH value (represented in part by urine pH) and the evaluation of the degree of excess protein is done rather quickly by measuring urine pH and using **darkfield microscopy**. Darkfield microscopy is a very quick investigative method, well suited to clinical practice, which yields information concerning the blood's buffer capacity, protein content and endobiontic infestation of the interstitial fluid and the blood cells. In addition, diversionary disturbances can be detected based on the symplasts and crystals present, as well as blockages of the leukocytes in cases of trace element deficiency, toxic burden or degenerative ten-dencies.

The experienced darkfield diagnostician can also recognize the endobiontic stress of the blood and the consequent therapeutic urgency (see table: Significance of Darkfield Microscopy).

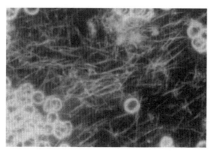 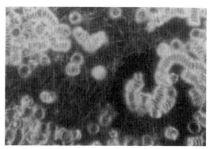

Figure A   Figure B

Figure A: "Hyperacidity" in the Darkfield: rapid filament formation, thick, bright Endobiont-burdened cell walls, high degenerative tendency.

Blood left standing has a tendency to form burr cells. High-valence Macrosymprotits.

Figure B: Excess protein in the Darkfield. Rouleau formation with thick protein edging all around, viscous movements; in thin smears "lemon-shaped" and "pear-shaped" erythrocyte formations.

Preparation left standing has a tendency to form long Chondrite snakes and Ascits. Symplast formation and protein crystals. The Symplasts are a sign that primarily diversion therapies and dietary measures must be instituted. Sickness of overproteinization are chronic diseases, generally develop slowly and massively interfere with cellular and eliminatory metabolism.

Hyperproteinemia of the organism, especially of the interstices, leads to decreased mitochondrial activity – i.e. cellular respiration – and thus to increased degenerative tendency of the cells and tissues. It must therefore always be dealt with on the cellular level, which means stimulating respiratory enzymes and treating the interstitial space.

Physiological protein decomposition mechanisms
Cellular incorporation and restructuring of protein in enzymes, etc.: 40 g (1.3 oz.)/day. Any excess supply must be excreted, broken down or stored: physiological breakdown of proteins takes place by way of purine synthesis, as protein is decomposed to amino acids. Purines are excreted as uric acid. This breakdown mechanism is highly acidic.

But excretion of excess protein also puts a burden on the eliminatory metabolism. Normally, in the steady state, about 40 g (1.3 oz.) of proteins are excreted daily as waste products, free radicals and toxins. The eliminatory mechanism is thus at times working at full capacity. If additional proteins (our daily average of 50-100 g (1.6-3.2 oz.) must be excreted, then the eliminatory mechanisms will be forced to work at overcapacity, leading to purine elimination pathologies: the body is then only partially equipped to deal with the excess protein elimination and therefore takes some metabolic shortcuts.

Increased uric acid production: uric acid is not very soluble. A great deal of fluid needs to be drunk, or else uric acid crystals will form in the tissues. These can also be detected (using Darkfield microscopy) in the blood as minuscule, sharp-edged, very geometric crystals. These uric acid crystals are seen as foreign bodies, they have a mechanical scrubbing effect and can trigger the clinical picture of acute gout.

The therapy for elevated uric acid production consists of drinking more fluids and stimulating kidney activity with Solidago, Berberis, diuretic teas and a strict low-protein diet. Administering xanthinoxidase hammers (e.g. Allopurinal/Zyloric) is not recommended, since this overburdens other pathological purine excretory pathways without getting rid of the basic problem. Amino acid deposits are dealt with by the latent hyperacidity: the negatively charged amino acids bind with minerals, leading to a lack of available minerals and to calcium complex depositions in the tissues.

Typically, the long-term hyperproteinated patient exhibits, on the one hand, mineral deficiency in bone and cartilage and, on the other, calcification in the soft tissues. The skin of such patients is thickened, large-pored, increasingly light sensitive and – especially on the seborrheal parts of the face, cheeks and chest – reddened. These patients tend to be "allergic to the sun".

The Significance of Proteins and Hyperproteinemia
The adult body needs about 40 grams (1.3 oz.) of pure protein daily to maintain metabolic equilibrium (harmonious balance of protein anabolism and catabolism); this amounts to 0.5-0.7 gram per kilogram (0.008-0.011 ounces/pound) of body weight. Daily consumption is about

EXCESS PROTEIN			
Protein Metabolism Statistics from Europe			
Consumption:	maximum	70 grams/day	(2.3 oz.)
Intake:	actual	120-150 grams/day	(4-5 oz.)
Intake:	ideal	40-70 grams/day	(1.3-2.3 oz.)
ELIMINATORY PATHWAYS			
Metabolism:	breakdown amino acids → purine → uric acid glyconeogenesis		
Elimination:	kidneys: ±0! liver: 10-40 grams/day (0.3-1.3 oz.) toxicity skin menstrual periods!		
Deposits:	• Blood BP↑-O₂↑ • Tissue • Interstitium (Pischinger) • Connective tissue rigidity		

60 grams (2 oz.) daily, keeping in mind that part of the catabolized cell protein can be recycled in the form of amino acids and a small portion converted to glucose (see below, gluconeogenesis) or used in hormone conversion.

Animal proteins are better absorbed in the small intestine, since they stimulate higher levels of hormone secretion and hydrochloric acid production. They are therefore highly praised by the meat industry. However, this ignores the fact that the only good aspect is its absorption; it is inferior when it comes to being incorporated or modified in body cells. Animal proteins – especially pork – are taken up and stored in the interstitium as higher molecular forms, peptides or low-molecular-weight proteins.

Plant proteins are decomposed into smaller components (amino acids) in the intestinal tract and then absorbed into the body. These amino acids, especially the essential amino acids, are easier for the cells to incorporate. It has thus been able to be demonstrated that plant proteins can be used to a much greater degree for cell construction, especially muscle cells.

Large-scale sports medicine studies have established that a strict vegetarian diet and the regular training regimen led to markedly superior endurance compared to an animal protein diet. In particular, it turned out that a vegetarian diet was able to improve cellular respiration (i.e. a mitochondrial function).

The mean per capita daily protein intake in Germany and Switzerland is about 140 grams (4.6 oz.)/day. Since the optimum amount that can be processed is 40-60 grams (1.3-2 oz.) of protein daily, the excess protein amounts to 50-100 grams (1.6-3.2 oz.) daily per person! This surplus protein cannot be processed in the cells and must either be decomposed, oxidized or stored in the body (see the work of Wendt). Amino acids and small protein molecules carry a negative charge and tend to combine with positively charged minerals. This results in chemically inert, nearly unreactive protein-mineral complexes with an extremely high tendency to deposit in the interstitium and tissues (see below: degenerative tendency). These protein accumulations lead to a diminution of tissue responsiveness, interstitial "clogging" and an alteration of the normal state of the interstitial fluid. The interstitium, which is an information carrier and the medium of all material exchange, becomes less able to carry out its transport function, which leads in turn to flooding of the tissues and cells with toxins and the deposition of metabolites in the interstitium.

A simple comparison can help one understand these burdensome processes: a bricklayer is building a house and can process a ton of bricks per day. If he is kept adequately supplied, he can work at maximum capacity. But if he gets 2 tons of bricks delivered every day, he must spend a certain portion of his working hours stacking and storing the surplus bricks. His daily output will thus be reduced. If this oversupply condition lasts very long, then the storage area will grow to be so large that it will further limit his ability to perform his duties. In the end, the bricklayer will be entirely occupied with stacking and storing the excess building materials, which finally collapse around him and totally prevent him from doing his work. Both the bricklayer (the analogue of the body's metabolism) and the building (the organs) suffer or are destroyed.

Gluconeogenesis: In case of emergency, human metabolism can turn to an energy-producing mechanism called gluconeogenesis. During hungry times, glucose can be extracted from proteins, as they get broken down and re-formed into glucose. This anaerobic form of energy production is accompanied by lactate formation, which is acidic and thus favors high-valence forms of the *Mucor racemosus* cycle. *Mucor racemosus* develops upward in a lactate-rich environment (Enderlein – Bacterial Cyclogeny). In patients with excess protein, this leads to overburdening with glucose and hence to hyperinsulinism and – paradoxically – also to increased hunger sensation. For this reason, we recommend, for patients with excess protein, on the one hand an animal-protein-free diet and on the other abstention from sugar consumption entirely. By means of gluconeogenesis, up to 40 grams (1.3 oz.) of protein daily can be broken down – although, as pointed out above, only by imposing a severe burden on the pancreas and liver due to new glycogen formation.

Prostaglandin synthesis: (see diagram) Prostaglandins are albuminous substances that are synthesized in the body as by products of cellular catabolism and as a breakdown product of arachidonic acid. The body

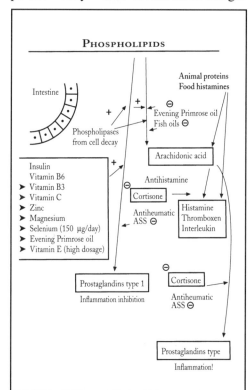

PHOSPHOLIPIDS

Intestine

Phospholipases from cell decay

Animal proteins
Food histamines

Evening Primrose oil
Fish oils ⊖

Arachidonic acid

Insulin
Vitamin B6
➤ Vitamin B3
➤ Vitamin C
➤ Zinc
➤ Magnesium
➤ Selenium (150 µg/day)
➤ Evening Primrose oil
➤ Vitamin E (high dosage)

Antihistamine

Cortisone

Antirheumatic
ASS ⊖

Histamine
Thromboxen
Interleukin

Prostaglandins type 1
Inflammation inhibition

Cortisone

Antirheumatic
ASS ⊖

Prostaglandins type
Inflammation!

receives arachidonic acid only as a nutritional component of animal-based foods; it is not found in plant-based foods.

As can be seen in the diagram, the body's prostaglandin synthesis can be shifted in favour of type I prostaglandins (which inhibit inflammation) by administering antioxidants, vitamins, evening primrose oil and selenium. Arachidonic acid from animal dietary components, however, is always metabolized to type II prostaglandins, which promote inflammations. At the same time, the formation of histamines, inflammation parameters and thromboxane is stimulated, which explains the elevated tendency to allergies and thromboses of those with animal-protein diets.

Most anti-inflammatories, as well as cortisone, have an inhibitory effect on the formation of type I & II prostaglandins and lead to arachidonic acid congestion, which in its turn leads to increased interleukin and thromboxane synthesis and to an increased tendency to inflammation after discontinuing cortisone or anti-inflammatory medication. This metabolic mechanism also explains the elevated leukocyte count (and the greater tendency to thromboses) during longer-term steroid therapy. Therefore, an animal-protein-free diet is very important in cases of hyperproteinemia, as is treatment with anti-oxidants, particularly vitamins E, C and evening primrose oil (see Lancet 1991, "Vegetarian Diet for Rheumatoid Arthritis"). Additional metabolic pathways for protein elimination: Metabolism of proteins takes place mainly in the liver. The metabolic capacity is about 40 grams (1.3 oz.) per day in healthy adults – from which it is clear that the liver is pretty much fully occupied in maintaining the metabolic balance if it is overseeing the process of the physiological conversion of 40 grams (1.3 oz.) of protein daily.

If, in addition, excess proteins flushed out of the interstices have to be processed, then, over the long term, the liver becomes overburdened, leading to toxin reflux. Most toxins are proteins, often structures of high molecular weight. The body then attempts to return them to storage or to excrete them via the skin. Toxins can also function as free radicals, increasing the body's oxidative tendency, and they can also be carcinogens. The attempt to excrete toxins via the skin leads to the skin changes mentioned above, with a tendency to skin inflammations and the deposition of free radicals in the skin. The consequences are pigment disorders, susceptibility to skin cancer and skin eczemas.

Another very important pathway for protein excretion is menstruation. The monthly elimination of 100-300 ml (3-10 oz.) of mostly coagulated blood represents a significant diversion of toxins and proteins. For women, this is a very important detoxification process. It also explains why women, during their menstruation years, exhibit fewer degenerative and civilization-induced diseases than men and why, after menopause, they begin catching up to the men in this respect. From our biological-holistic point of view, therefore, these monthly periods represent a very effective detoxification procedure, and we are strongly against the liberal diagnosis of hysterectomy before menopause. From a holistic point of view, the quite common myomas among middle-aged women are also merely an expression of hyperproteinemia and protein deposits between the muscle cells, and can be successfully treated, locally and systemically, with diversion therapy and Mucor therapy.

Additional Hyperproteinemia Diseases
Non-metabolized proteins can affect the organism via two pathophysiological mechanisms:

1. Increased dissolution in the interstitial spaces and circulatory systems: as described above, the permeability of soluble substances in the interstices is inversely proportional to the protein content. Water's ability to act as an information carrier is dependent on its purity. Thus, the transport of substances in the blood – but especially in the interstices – is lowered by a high protein content, which compromises cellular respiration. The consequence is an elevated degenerative tendency (premature cell aging and degeneration). Protein-free fasting thus reduces the degenerative tendency and promotes the detoxification of the organism – which is why fasting has been recommended as far back as the Old Testament and in ancient healing systems.

2. In the blood, hyperproteinemia lowers the ability to take up oxygen. Erythrocytes usually carry a positive surface charge and repel each other due to this electrostatic like charge, freeing up their entire functional

surface. If there are amino acids and low-molecular-weight proteins dissolved in the blood, which always have a negative valence, then these unite with the erythrocytes, binding them into protein-covered chains (rouleau formation), which only possess a limited capacity to take up oxygen. This rouleau formation in turn favours degenerative tendencies and can be detected quickly and easily in the Darkfield microscope.

Darkfield Microscopy therefore allows a very quick milieu diagnosis, recognition as to which therapeutic approaches are the most urgent, e.g. the necessity of deproteinization.

The consequences of rouleau and conglomerate formation of erythrocytes are thromboses, lowered oxygen intake, microembolisms and circulatory disorders. Tissue cells are inadequately supplied with oxygen and become anoxic, making anaerobic energy production necessary. This (glycolysis) creates lactate and promotes the growth of higher *Mucor racemosus* valences. This explains the statement frequently encountered in the lay literature, that excess protein and/or animal protein causes the endobiosis. But it also means that patients with the consequent symptoms of cellular respiration, such as coronary heart disease, circulatory disorders, hypertonia, etc. usually have a Mucor endobiosis, and that its vicious cycle can be broken with Mucokehl and respiratory-chain enzymes (Sanuvis).

Hypertonia is explicable in the same manner, and can usually be normalized with long-term deproteinization, alkaline therapy and treatment with Sanuvis (lactic acid) and Mucokehl *(Mucor racemosus)*. Hypertonic patients very frequently exhibit rouleau formation in a Darkfield examination. In the therapy test, a very satisfactory breakdown of the rouleau formations can be noted after administration of Mucokehl. The blood's reduced oxygen-carrying capacity is compensated by attempting to improve circulation by raising the blood pressure. Hypertonia thus represents, in our view, an attempt to compensate a reduced oxygen uptake capacity of the blood in vivo.

3.   If hyperproteinemia persists for longer periods, the body attempts to bind the pathological negative valences with positively charged minerals, resulting in the formation of nearly insoluble mineral-protein complexes (calcification). The sclerotic build-ups and deposits in vessels and tissues

lead to a reduction in organ function, additional reduction of material supply to tissues and to the well-known late complications of vascular rigidity (arteriosclerosis). Additional complications will be treated in the section "Consequences of Latent Hyperacidity".

Treating Hyperproteinemia

Hyperproteinemia therapy must always proceed in parallel with hyperacidity therapy, and must also treat the consequences of reduced cellular respiration and Endobiontic infestation, otherwise the vicious cycle cannot be interrupted. Treating hyperproteinemia is a long-term therapy, usually lasting for years and requiring a change in life-style, especially dietary habits. A thoroughly administered hyperproteinemia therapy is at the same time the best preventive measure against degenerative ailments and malignant diseases.

Fasting is quite often a good beginning to treating excess protein. However, one needs to keep in mind that, first of all, the excretory mechanisms are often already overburdened and that a waste product attack is possible. This can quickly and easily be checked using Darkfield Microscopy:

- Are there rouleau formations?

- Are there symplasts (indicate over-burdened protein processes)?

- Are there crystals (indicate long-term hyperproteinemia)?

Werthmann and Rau's Hypoallergenic Diet
Forbidden: Cow's milk and all dairy products: Yoghurt, cottage cheese, ice cream, chocolate, cheese and cheese dishes. Nuts and nut dishes, Chicken, eggs and egg dishes, cakes, etc. Pork and ham, sausages. Citrus fruits (all fruits in the evening). All histamine-rich meats, rabbit, venison, and anchovies
Permitted: All vegetables, potatoes, chestnuts, fruit, rice, soya dishes, grain dishes; veal, chicken and fish (only once a week)

In addition, it is necessary to keep in mind that fasting must never become starvation, because metabolic processes slow down when the organism is starving, which, for patients suffering from excess protein, is precisely what one would like at all costs to avoid. Therefore, one must supply the body with certain substances, which without presenting a burden, help to ensure enzymatic activity and metabolic functions. We therefore usually combine fasting therapy with enzyme therapy and neural therapy of the excretory organs as well as the thyroid gland. Later on, the fasting phase needs to transition into an animal-protein-free diet, or one very low in animal protein.

The diet should initially as free from animal protein as possible, including dairy products. This is not the place to go into the many and frequent combinations of hyperproteinemia and food allergies, but we do recommend – because of the commonness of dairy allergies – a hypoallergenic diet at first (as described by Werthmann and Rau), which is both very alkaline and rich in trace elements.

A hypoallergenic diet enables (for those many food allergy sufferers) a build-up of the mucosa of the small intestine and thereby improved digestion of dietary protein. Alkaline foods are recommended: almost all vegetables, fruits (eaten in the morning), potatoes, chestnuts, corn (See "How can I Eat a Properly Acid-Base Balanced Diet?" R. Bircher-Ray, Humata Verlag).

Alkaline therapy – two starting points:

A) Providing base-equivalents

B) Replacing and providing positively-charged trace elements, minerals and electrolytes

As regards A) above: in the majority of cases, alkaline therapy can be administered orally; by dint of long-term (a year or more) provision of base equivalents, it effects a neutralization of excess acidic deposits in the tissues. The alkaline orientation promotes the organism's constructive powers, as can be seen in the physiological alkalinity of small children. Any shift in the acidic direction encourages sclerotic and degenerative tendencies in the organism.

The alkaline supply is in the form of Alkala N. This must be administered during the day, at a time when no digestive activity is going on or imminent. It can thus be taken very early in the morning, but physiologically best around 10 AM or 4 PM, when the body has its normal alkaline episodes (absorption of the bicarbonate secreted by the pancreas). Alkala dosage: 2½ measuring spoons dissolved in 20-30 cc (7-10 oz.) of water.

In cases of strong degenerative tendency, much filament formation in the Darkfield or pronounced symptoms of hyperacidity, we administer the alkaline therapy parenterally; the dosage normally amounts to 500 ml (17 oz.) of the Paracelsus Alkaline Solution 1-2 times weekly, into which we also mix the diversion agents and catalysts mentioned below.

As an alternative to Alkala, we have – much like the alkaline mixtures of the F.X. Mayr physicians – created an alkaline solution which is at the same time a mineral therapy and which, because of the orotic acid (magnesium orotate), promotes cellular respiration. But it is of utmost importance that alkaline therapy be carried out in concert with a change in dietary habits and on a long-term basis. Initial flatulence when taking Alkala is an indication of excess hydrochloric acid in the stomach, which is being neutralized by Alkala through the formation of CO_2. This problem generally only lasts a few days, and this is why Alkala should be taken on an empty stomach. Sometimes the patient might have diarrhoea at the beginning; this indicates an overly acid milieu in the small intestine, which likewise normalizes out after a few days (and, incidentally, strongly confirms the necessity of Alkala therapy).

4. Diversion Therapy

All excretory organs should be activated by improving circulation (exercise, heat applications, reflex applications such as cupping massages, neural therapy, etc.). Liver activity is stimulated by means of bile-activating and liver-cell-activating therapeutic agents: Liv 52 (Ayurmedica), Hepar comp. (Heel), Taraxacum, Chelidonium, wormwood tea, etc. The kidneys are stimulated with Solidago, Betula, drinking lots of fluids.

5. Stimulating Cellular Respiration

Aerobic energy production in the mitochondria is stimulated by highly dilute dextrorotary lactic acid (Sanuvis) or citric acid (Citrokehl). For Mucor types, Sanuvis is usually more effective; for Aspergillus types, who are susceptible to tubercular maladies, Citrokehl is usually more suitable. Here, too, a longer-term treatment is important and reinforces the isopathic therapy considerably. We have also had good results with the "catalysts of the citric acid cycle", with quinones and with coenzymes, particularly coenzyme Q10 (found in ubiquinone), coenzyme comp. (Heel) and similar preparations.

Orthomolecular Therapy/ Trace Element Substitution

Supplying positively-charged valences in the form of trace elements is extremely important. Chronic hyperacidity leads, as described above, to a trace element deficiency and binding of the trace elements. The binding sites of the trace elements are then no longer occupied and pathological, toxic elements such as mercury, cadmium and lead take the place of selenium, zinc and magnesium. This relative and absolute trace element deficiency explains the very high incidence of heavy-metal toxicity. Therefore, the trace elements selenium, zinc and magnesium must be substituted over the long term. For the initial evaluation, we use hair mineral analyses, which have proven themselves better than serum analyses. Administering the trace elements is done materially and informatively, i.e. with orthomolecular dosages and homeopathic preparations. This way, the body is supplied, on the one hand, with the building materials it needs and, on the other, the homeopathics probably improve, informatively, its uptake into the cells.

Our recommended daily dosage is: selenium 150 micrograms, zinc 15 mg, manganese 5 mg. Manganese is an especially important trace element and catalyzes various enzymatic processes which are important in protein metabolism and energy production. For similar reasons, we also substitute chromium with a dosage of 100-200 micrograms per day. Chromium is especially essential to the pancreas and hence for the synthesis of proteases, so important in processing excess protein.

Isopathic Therapy using Sanum Preparations

The diseases of modern life on the one hand and of the tubercular maladies on the other are the primary areas of application of isopathic agents. Depending on place and localization, as well as the patient's constitution, hyperproteinemia promotes the upward development of the higher endobiontic valences. The Endobiont infestation in turn increases cell-wall rigidity and with it the degenerative trend. Therefore, Darkfield

---

HYPERACIDITY

Intracellular pH 7.28-7.45
Causes of Acidity
Endogenous   • Intestinal fermentation → lactic acid
                   • Weak stomach function
Exogenous   • Hypoalkalinity/minerals
                   • Excess protein
                         Amino Acids
                   • Glycolysis
                   • Lipocatabolism → ketones
                   • Stress

THE SYMPTOMS OF HYPERACIDITY
Organs which express hyperacidity

Kidney/Bladder	cystitis/prostate genital fungi
Stomach	hyperacidity
Skin	sweating allergies, "toxic" reaction eczemas
Intestines	acid stools, colitis
Bronchia	pressure hyperactive bronchia asthma
Joints	myalgia arthritis

examinations mostly turn up erythrocytes with a strong intracellular Endobiont infestation (sporoid Symprotits and brightly-lit wall thickenings). These changes point to a very high degenerative tendency and are practically always seen in carcinoma cases. Long-term therapy with Mucokehl *(Mucor racemosus)*, or possibly Mucokehl alternating with Nigersan *(Aspergillus niger)*, is thus necessary. For circulatory diseases of civilization, we recommend at least a one-year treatment period of 2-3 tablets of Mucokehl daily, taken mornings and evenings, and 1-2 tablets of Nigersan every evening. In cases involving severe congestive problems, we recommend administering Sanuvis for the same period, 30-50 drops thrice daily. Diet and concomitant therapy with Alkala during the entire term of therapy are a must. One should inform the patient that this treatment generally takes several weeks before it improves the patient's subjective condition, and that complaints such as angina pectoris, hypertonia, dizziness and suchlike usually abate quite considerably within a few months. For patients with severe hyper-proteinemia, chronic inflammation or extensive rou-leau formation, I recommend an extra enzyme therapy in the initial phase (Wobenzym or Phlogenzym), starting at a high dosage level and decreasing gradually. Patients often find this treatment to be very pleasant.

The Clinical Picture of Hyperacidity

The overall human metabolism is slightly acidic, due to the endo-genous production of acids (see diagram). The intracellular pH value is weakly basic in the range 7.28-7.45. In order to maintain this weak basic value, acid must continually be eliminated in the urine, which is why the mean urine pH value is markedly lower. Urine pH varies, with two daily basic peak values. This occurs because, some time after eating, excess bicarbonate pro-duced by the pancreas is absorbed in the small intestine. We support this physiological mechanism by stimulating the pancreas (chromium doses, Fortakehl *(Penicillium roquefortii)*, pancreatric preparations, Leptandra, etc.) and by administering Alkala N or some other alkaline agent during digestion-free times, i.e. around 10 AM and 4 PM.

The origin of the acids is shown in the diagram. Of importance are the connections with **intestinal fermentation**, which occurs as a result of excessive sugar supply – but also as a result of eating fruit in the evening – leads to lactate formation, which is strongly acidic. The lactate then promotes Mucor growth and glycolysis and hence degenerative tendencies in the organism. Eating fruit in the evening thus promotes acidity, since the pancreas produces fewer saccharases at night, so that the sugars released by the fruit are not absorbed, but instead glycolyzed and fermented by the intestinal flora. In the case of exogenous acid attacks, the two main causes are

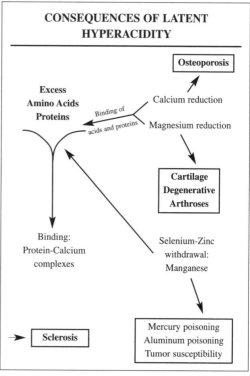

excessive amino-acid supply (proteins, see above) and reduced mineral supply.

Mechanisms for acid elimination: in order to maintain a steady acid-base equilibrium, the body needs to eliminate the acids produced by metabolic processes. Normally, this occurs via the kidneys, as acid urine is excreted at night and neutral urine during the day. If acid production or supply increases, the urine must be made correspondingly more acidic and the physiological alkaline urine periods drop out. The constantly acidic urine then can cause mucous membrane irritation, chronic cystitis and genital infection, as well as genital fungal infections and, in men, subliminal chronic prostate irritation. Every one of these ailments responds very well to thoroughly-administered alkaline therapy. In particular, frequently recurring cystitis in older female patients can be cured within a year without recourse to antibiotics.

If the kidneys are overburdened in their eliminatory function – which will show up as a constant highly acidic urine pH – then other eliminatory organs will be called on to help eliminate acids, which is then seen as a pH shift in perspiration, stool and bronchial secretion.

The **stomach** (a primary producer of acidity) reacts with hyperacidity, i.e. it secretes hydrochloric acid even at non-digestive times. This increased acid secretion leads to gastritis, then later on to ventricular or duodenal ulcers. However, elevated acid production is always an expression of the body's attempt to eliminate acid equivalents, and should therefore never be suppressed with hydrogen blockers, since then the equivalents which need to be eliminated remain in the body and lead to tissue acidosis and overtaxing of the blood's buffer mechanism.

Stomach hyperacidity can be eliminated in practically every case by long-term treatment with Alkala N and administration of minerals. The pancreas' bicarbonate production needs to be promoted (see above), for which we recommend the patient also take small doses of table salt (sodium chloride is needed in the synthesis of bicarbonate). Additionally, a strict animal-protein free diet must be maintained, since gastric acid and pepsin secretion is over stimulated by animal proteins.

The **skin** reacts to hyperacidity by secreting acidic perspiration. This, along with elevated perspiratory amino-acid elimination, leads to skin irritation, changes in skin pH and toxic skin reactions. Patients perspire more copiously and for no reason. Night sweats in particular are a classic sign of chronic acidity problems. (We have often observed, in menopausal female patients, quite a significant reduction of menopausal flush perspiration after dietary modification, administering minerals and Alkala therapy.)

Eczemas, allergic skin reactions and hypersensitive skin, are the consequences. In our view, every eczema patient is thus in need of an inner, systemic alkaline therapy, and an intestinal cleansing treatment must also be administered at the same time.

Intestines

The intestinal tract, the largest mucous membranal organ, is also the largest excretory organ. The secretions of the small intestine's mucous membrane amount to approximately 20 litres (4 gallons) per day, of which the major portion is re-absorbed in the ileum and the colon. The small intestinal mucus varies considerably in its acid content, ranging physiologically from pH 6.0-6.8 – from which it is clear that considerable acid excretion takes place in the small intestine. This needs to be neutralized by the chyme, which is why it is so important to ingest lots of minerals, as well as indigestible alkaline plant fibres. These neutralize intestinal acidity through the formation of phytates and other fibre complexes, which are then excreted in the stool.

If the intestine is not kept supplied with indigestible fibre (roughage), then acid is reabsorbed and the intestinal contents also become acidic, which can express itself as colitis and irritable colon. Colitis patients should therefore – most of the time gradually – switch over to an alkaline, fibre-rich, animal-protein-free diet. The very common food allergies (mostly milk proteins) must absolutely be taken into account as well, since all food allergies lead to atrophy of the small intestinal mucous membrane and thus to increased acid re-absorption.

Rhino-Bronchial System and the Lungs
The mucous membranes of the rhino-bronchial system can also be utilized for acid excretion. This then leads to increased bronchial secretion and viscous sinus mucus with a tendency to recurrent bronchitis or sinusitis. As indicated above, the viscosity of the mucus depends on the acid content. The consequences of these bronchial mucous changes include a **hyper-reactive bronchial tree and a tendency to asthma**. The patients often experience thoracic pressure, and we have also often noted mental and emotional symptoms as expressions of "hyperacidity". These manifest themselves as dejection, depression, obsessive recurrent thoughts and/or sleep disturbances. We therefore treat all patients with emotional symptoms by treating the inner milieu, regulation of the acid-base equilibrium and orthomolecular substitution.

Joints: joints have a serous skin and secrete inwards. When the endothelial-serous system is in acid-elimination mode, proteins, uric acid crystals and other acid equivalents are released into the joint, triggering inflammatory-reactions. A Darkfield examination of arthrocentesis fluid therefore shows mostly high-valence endobiontic structures and rapid development of coarse filaments as well as various crystalline structures – all of which express the acidity of the milieu. Correspondingly, inflammatory arthritis responds well to instillation with a sodium carbonate solution, Notakehl *(Penicillium notatum)* and Citrokehl (citric acid) for de-acidification. But the joints and connective tissue are also involved via the process of acid-induced decalcification and demineralization, which takes place in order to mobilize minerals and bind excess proteins. One therefore encounters, as a consequence of latent hyperacidity, de-calcification in the bones on the one hand and calcium deposits in the muscles, connective tissue, joint capsules and tissues on the other.

Further consequences of latent hyperacidity are described in the table above. Deprivation of cationic trace elements (selenium, zinc, manganese, calcium, magnesium) leads to osteoporosis, cartilage degeneration, trace element deficiency. The bonding sites which this process makes available can then be occupied by toxic trace elements and heavy metals, which is why mercury poisoning, aluminium poisoning and lead poisoning can have significantly stronger effects. This toxicity must therefore always be treated with deacidification. Thus, osteoporosis is not a calcium disorder, but rather a problem with excess protein, hyperacidity and bone-marrow metabolism, which can also be treated accordingly and which responds well to Sanum therapy and to improvement of bone-marrow metabolism: Latensin *(Bacillus cereus)*, Mucokehl *(Mucor racemosus)* and Nigersan *(Aspergillus niger)*/Citrokehl (citric acid), Alkala, Calcium fluoratum Injeel

Dr. Thomas Rau, M.D.
Paracelsus Klinik Lustmühle,
9062 Lustmühle (bei St.Gallen)
Switzerland

Published in Explore! Volume 6 Number 6 1996

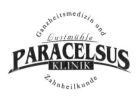

3

Some thoughts on the connection between Biological Medicine and Single Remedy Homoeopathy

In certain homoeopathic circles, the opinion still prevails that single remedy homoeopathy can not or does not need to be combined with other naturopathic therapies. In particular, it is thought useless and even wrong to administer trace-elements, to make acid/alkaline changes or take other energetic measures as an accompanying or a preventative therapy.

In contrast, based on our experience of many years, homoeopathic single remedies rarely develop their maximum therapeutic strength nowadays. On the other hand, patients react much better to homeopathic remedies straight after a previous milieu or Sanum therapy. In the following article, I try to explain this modern phenomenon of Homoeopathy and Isopathy:

Internal environment, feelings and homoeopathic repertoires:
With the determination of the correct homoeopathic treatment, the patient is "repertoireized", i.e. based on answers to the many questions put to him about his character and symptoms, the patient is assigned to a particular constitution-type. The answers to the questions are shaped by the present feelings and symptoms of the patient. In our experience however, people's feelings are fundamentally different with a changed internal milieu and/or with a toxic load, than in health. The symptoms are experienced differently.

If for example, the patient undergoes an anti-acid therapy, then he feels differently afterwards, more peaceful and not as "sour"!

Thus, after a milieu therapy, one assigns the patients to another constitution-type than before the milieu therapy. In other words: only after a milieu therapy can the correct remedy be found, which then works thoroughly, since the milieu therapy also improves regulation and reaction.

An attempt at a physical explanation of Homoeopathy and Milieu Therapy:

The effect of homoeopathic single remedies, in dilutions of over D30, is not material, since usually no more molecules of the active substance are present in them but they have a fine-energetic informative effect on the carrier substances of the mesenchyme. In particular, one assumes that water molecules bound in the mesenchyme and arranged along polysaccharide molecules, are changed in their form. These water molecules are not however present in single molecules, but rather in the form of spatially, specially arranged groups of molecules, so-called cluster-molecules. This cluster-molecule formation is a peculiarity of the element water, which probably explains a majority of its special characteristics.

With laser spectrographic and photon emission analyses, molecules and their changes, as well as the energy emission of substances, can be measured. From such investigations, it is well-known that homeopathica affect the cluster-structures of the water-molecule connections, in particular their spherical angular arrangement. It could be proven that water molecules arrange themselves in groups, in a spatial arrangement of approx. 15 – 25 molecules. These groups of molecules (called clusters) can take up, by nature of their spatial arrangement, other molecules and electrons, temporarily bind and then release them. They thereby act as transporters and also have the possibility of changing their electron and photon emission.

If water changes into a gaseous condition, or if it is broken up by special methods (Levitation after Hacheney or special sprayings on stone), the molecule cluster becomes smaller, to the size of a single molecule or small cluster of 4 – 5 water molecules. The same takes place during manual homoeopathic shaking, which exposes the water to large forces of rotation and retardation. The smaller the clusters are, the more fine-energetic information (electrons and photons) can be bound to the molecular structures (= higher potencies). Levitated water or water from rushing, stone-rich brooks is thus more able to exchange or take up information. This ability of the water molecules to change, probably explains the entire information exchange quality of the mesenchyme, and thus the interstitial area (Pischinger area).

Mesenchyme, acidity and protein condition:

Additionally, high-molecular polysaccharide molecules exist in the mesenchyme, the actual workshop of homoeopathica, which are geometrically aligned, at normal pH (acidity), parallel to each other. Substances are transported along them and following their charge, in particular if they also have a charge and are thus not inert materials. Water molecule clusters are thus also better or less well transported, according to their added electrons or bound molecules. Information exchange in the mesenchyme thus depends on the polysaccharide structure and the electromagnetic charge and/or the electrical resistance potential of the mesenchyme. However, these factors depend again on the redox potential of a liquid, the electrical resistance and also the pH value.

If too many free H+ ions are in the mesenchyme, then the pH value is too sour and the polysaccharide molecules arrange themselves into interlaced and chaotic forms. If too many free, metabolized protein molecules are present (over-acidification), then the conductivity in the mesenchyme also decreases.

The adaptability of an organism and its internal transport ability are thus based on the intactness of the mesenchymal liquid.

The influence of the environment on the homoeopathic constitution:

It is now well-known that especially environmental factors have a large influence on the interstitial area and the ability of water to exchange information. Both proteins and heavy metals, with their positive surface charges, bind themselves almost irreversibly to the mesenchymal structures and thus change the electromagnetic surface tension and electrical charge of these mesenchymal molecules. As already described in Hahnemann's times, mercury works particularly strongly in blocking lymph activity, in the same way that proteins, because of their ability to load and unload H+ ions, can block mesenchymal activity. The consequences of such environment loads, is the fact that the information receptiveness and the material transfer ability of the mesenchyme are decreased or lost. The patient is therefore less accessible for informative, single remedy homoeopathic and other energetic therapies.

Clinical experience shows that effectiveness of information therapies is considerably improved by mesenchymal pre-treatments like milieu therapy, orthomolecular therapy, acid-alkaline balancing and Isopathy. Because of their heavy metal and protein overload, today's patients react poorly, if at all, to single remedy homeopathy or information therapies, but that the effectiveness of such therapies can massively be improved by a milieu therapy over many months .

That is why it is important, before a single remedy homeopathy treatment, for the patient to be pre-treated with orthomolecular therapy, Isopathy and acid-alkaline balancing.

Some elements which work particularly well to prepare the patients for Homeopathica, are minerals, salts and metals, in material concentrations: magnesium, orotic acid, silicon, potassium, manganese and molybdenum, as well as potassium and, in rarer cases, calcium.

Particularly worth mentioning is the orthomolecular influence of magnesium (sympathetic reduction) on the parasympathetic nervous system and potassium (parasympathetic reinforcement), which favors the fine-regulation and improves the effectiveness of homeopathica.

Also worth mentioning are catalytic substances such as zinc as well as organic substances such as Acidum phosphoricum, Chinone, etc. which already occur in homoeopathic concentrations in normal cell metabolism and have with certainty an interaction with single remedy homeopathy. Again, it becomes clear how strongly cell metabolism affects each homeopathic therapy.

Teeth, heavy metals and internal environment – The meaning of regulation blockades:

In order for a homeopathic therapy to work, the body needs the ability to react and to convert fine-energetic stimulations. This ability to react is called "regulation" in biological medicine. This refers to a transfer of information at a very basic level: the recognizing of a stimulation and its focused conversion into a tissue reaction

So-called "regulation blockades", which play an enormous role in biological medicine, can suppress this ability to regulate. Patients with regulation blockades cannot react to fine homeopathic attractions. High potency homeopathica will only work if the blockades are eliminated:

The most frequent regulation blockades are:
- Heavy metals (most frequent sources: fillings and artificial denture materials, which contain mercury or palladium. These highly toxic heavy metals are taken up in the body and have there a long-term effect, obstructing very many important chemical metabolic reactions. They work as antagonists to the important trace elements, e.g. zinc, selenium or manganese.
- Dead teeth and concentrations of bacterial ostitis in the jaw: each root treated tooth is a dead tooth and carries highly toxic poisons in the mesenchyme / lymph. Additionally, each root treated tooth is bacterially infected and these bacteria have a blocking influence on the immune system and the associated meridian and its organs.
- Dysbiosis of the intestines (= incorrect intestinal bacteria): The intestinal bacteria are our main detoxer and protect against other pathological bacteria. With the absence of the normal bacteria, pathological bacteria and intestinal flora arise, which freely distribute toxins.
- Lack of trace elements
- Over-acidification and protein overload
- Continuous psychological stress
- Chemical effects such as antiphlogistica, steroids, etc..

The importance of complex homoeopathica:
The realization that homoeopathica work better, if blockades are eliminated at the same time, induced the founder of homotoxikologie, the important homoeopath Dr. med. Hans Heinrich Reckweg, to place homoeopathica together which, on the one hand, contain the classical homoeopathic substances and on the other hand, encourage the processes of cell-metabolism.

These substances are the so-called chinones and catalysts of the citrus acid cycle. In addition, Dr. Reckweg began to combine homeopathic substances with homeopathically treated remedies which aimed at energizing certain organs of elimination and thus to improve the effectiveness of the low-potency homeopathica. The third group of substances, which were likewise combined with conventional homoeopathica, are the cell-preparations, which have an energizing effect on organ activities. These are homoeopathica, that are won from cell material from the organs of healthy young animals.

The combination of these different homeopathic groups results in complex preparations, which are called "complex homoeopathica". These substance combinations have organotropic effects and are outstanding supplements for milieu therapy.

They have, in contrast to single remedy homeopathy, less an effect on the basic nature and archetypal themes of a patient's life than metabolic and eliminating processes. They also in no way compete with the high potency single remedy homeopathy, but prepare the body for the single remedies. For more information consult the text books on homotoxicology or the large Vademecum of the Heel company).

Internal milieu, feelings and psyche:
A completely new aspect, which is always neglected with homeopathic therapy, is the influence of the nature, mode of thought and the metabolic reactions of patients by changes in diet, detoxification and orthomolecular therapy. Patients, who are toxically loaded, have chronic viral infections and chronic mesenchymal clogging ("over-acidification"), think, feel and act differently than after a metabolic regeneration over many months. So the patient's "repertoireized" constitution is frequently not the true nature of the patient, which only reveals itself after a longer lasting milieu therapy. This explains why homeopathica so often don't work without a preceding milieu therapy, since the "wrong" constitution was being projected. Again and again I see in my practice that patients, just by making dietary changes or with an anti-acid therapy, gain access to their life's fundamental themes and their life situation and thus change their homoeopathic constitutional type.

This explains, from another side, that the profound homeopathic effect of single remedies only takes place after a milieu therapy body cleaning and metabolic adjustment.

Only after such a constitutional milieu retuning can the patient then be correctly "repertoireized".

A further paradigm of many homeopaths, is the exclusiveness with which pure homeopathy is postulated. No other supporting therapies are permitted, as if these could have an adverse effect on the correctly selected remedy! On the other hand however, manifested toxicities and blockades should not disturb, according to the opinion of the homeopath, e.g. arsenic in tooth root fillings, sulfur in pork, phosphor from organic acids, etc. etc.! Substances develop continually in the metabolism of the patient, which would also work as homeopathica, or even change homeopathic archetypes. Paradoxically, on the other hand, strict homeopaths warn again and again that peppermint blocks all homoeopathica, which may be partly correct but this exclusiveness is however nonsense. Mint contains etheric oils, saturated, long chain oils, as contained in many animal products but also in many aromatic substances.

Isn't it now evident, after all the above, that nutrition and the metabolic situation alone can have the strongest influence on the patient's constitution, as well as his basic nature and way of thinking and not be separated from homeopathic principles?

And what affect does it have when the patient eats large quantities of animal protein and thereby ingests the essential being of the tortured animals, their homeopathic constitution and their genetically altering endobiontic and viral loads? So the true homoeopath would nevertheless actually have to demand his patient to be purely natural, toxin free, and vegan!

It is thus important that it is finally recognized in single remedy homoeopathic circles that milieu therapy and orthomolecular medicine are the basis of biological medicine and that homoeopathica will only work, with their addition, in the sense of a crowning therapy. Still, I experience fantastic results in my practice with high potency homeopathic therapies. These are however individual cases, usually with pronounced constitutional situations. Broadly combined milieu therapies behave completely differently, with symptoms of approx. 80% of all chronic diseases strongly improving within 2–6 months. The combination of different biomedical methods with single remedy homeopathy is re the therapy of the our time, particularly if a dietary conversion, ense of vegetarian nutrition, and the appropriate conversion of the internal milieu of the patient takes place at the same time.

PRACTICAL SUGGESTIONS TO IMPROVEMENT OF MILIEU AND REGULATION:

Milieu therapy must always take place individually and esp. consider toxic conditions. The following prescriptions are only a general suggestion. Treatment should be carried out several weeks to months:

Improvement of the acid-alkaline environment:
- vegetarian food, no cow's milk products, no sugar
- drink large quantities, esp. warm water, 2 liters per day
- Alkala N 1–2 x daily ½ measuring spoon · Sanuvis drop (Lactovis®) 2–3 x 30 drops a day
- Mapurit (Sanum, 2 x 1 caps) or an other multi-mineral preparation

Heavy metal detox:
- selenium, 100–200mcgr/d, e.g. as Selenmethionin (2x1, Sanum) or Selenase
- vitamin C 1–2 gr/day for several months
- Ev.Bio Chlorella 2–3 x 4–6 tabl.

Intestinal flora regeneration and endobiontical environment:
- Sankombi drops 3 x 8–10 drops (Sanum),
- for Utilin D6 caps and Recarcin D6 caps, per a caps per week.

Improvement of "cell breathing": (esp. chron. and neurological suffering)
- Ubichinon comp.(Heel) 1 amp. s.c., twice per week or as nose therapy
- catalysts of the citric acid cycle (Heel), each 2. day an amp. or s.c. as described
- Coenzyme Q 10 90–120 mg daily

Dr. Thomas Rau, M.D.
Paracelsus Klinik Lustmühle,
9062 Lustmühle (bei St.Gallen)
Switzerland

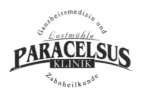

4

Milieu Therapy, Isopathy and Darkfield Microscopy: Connections with Holistic Dental Medicine

The concept of "blockades" or hindrances to healing

The most frequent hindrances to healing at the present time are, on the one hand, dental foci causing fields of interference and toxicity (i.e. mostly iatrogenic influences) and, on the other hand, dysbioses of the intestinal system with a consequent enterotoxic load. Hindrances to healing, the so-called "blockades", are indicated by a reduced ability to regulate, i.e. a reduction in the body's ability to react to external stimuli. Free radicals and persistent immune complexes develop, also accompanied by a reduction in the inflammatory response or "false" inflammations. As a result, toxic products are deposited and pathological protein structures, which Professor Enderlein named "endobiontic high valencies", build up in the body.

All these symptoms share the feature that protein structures, present in the body in a complex form with otherwise inert but toxic elements, bring the cells of the body into a state of impregnation and later degeneration. These materials lead to a false defensive reaction (auto-immune process) or to a flagging of the cell metabolism, i.e. to premature ageing or the growth of tumours. The cell metabolism decreases and the cells become degenerate.

Reasons for Sanum therapy

In the cells and in interstitial fluid, Sanum and milieu therapy offers a very effective solution to the change of protein structures and their dynamics and works on different levels:

The **orthomolecular substances** (trace elements, polyunsaturated fatty acids, stimulants such as citric or formic acid, vitamins) improve the cell metabolism, the membrane potential and thus the ability of the cells to react. The substances in this range include Alkala N, Lipiscor, Mapurit, Selenomethionine, Vitamin E Sanum, Formasan, Zinkokehl, Selenokehl, Cuprukehl, Citrokehl, and also substances such as evening primrose oil made by Biofrid.

The **acid base regulators** alter the permeability of the mesenchyme (embryonic connective tissue) and its ability to transport substances, and thus improve at a very fundamental level the ability of the body to regulate itself. They are complemented by a basic diet low in animal protein. New tests show that in the basic milieu the interstitial fluid from directed polysaccharide molecules is considerably better able to transport both material substances and exchange of energy. The substances in this range are: Alkala N and Alkala T, also the potency accords Sanuvis, Citrokehl and Formasan and indirectly the preparation Utilin S.

The **isopathic medications** show an ability to reduce high-molecular pathological protein structures ("endobiontic high valencies") and to prevent their upward development into microbiological structures such as viruses, bacteria or fungi. The medications are therefore also very effective in the area of the intestinal flora where they can lead to normalisation, provided that the patient sticks to a diet which will protect the intestinal flora – that is, without eggs, cow's milk products, sugar or meat.

SHORT DIGRESSION REGARDING THE PLEOMORPHISTIC APPROACH

According to Professor Dr. G. Enderlein, isopathic remedies reach deep into the metabolism and the inner milieu of the mesenchyme, the bodily fluids and the cells. At the root of them is pleomorphistic thinking which says that people and all animals are very intensely bound together with nature in their rhythm and reactions and that there is constant change (pleo = many, morph = form).

Bacteria are not "fixed units" which always develop the same illness, but they continually change – that is, they can metamorphose from one form into another and even become other bacteria or move into a fungal phase, the so-called "culmination" of the cycle of development. There are however also "viral" phases of the "symbiont" named below, and these develop upwardly both inside and outside the cells and have a direct influence on the metabolism of the cell. In molecular biology the jump from the double helix structure of acidic DNA to the double protein chain structure described by Enderlein has not yet been completely researched. However, the results achieved by researchers in Vienna are interesting: they have analysed the "protite" described by Enderlein as being identical to the globin of the haemoglobin, and because of this there was shown to be the closest possible link between human erythrocyte cells and the basic components of bacteria – those very bacteria which humans have in billions as symbionts on their skin, in the bowel and on all the mucous membranes, proving how closely the world of bacteria is tied up with the intact human organism.

However, the pleomorphists (Béchamp, von Brehmer, Enderlein and others) also describe "blood parasitism", i.e. the presence of the early stages of symbiontic bacteria. Enderlein called them "endobionts": they exist in the blood and all bodily fluids and can also be seen using darkfield microscopy. They can change pleomorphically from one form into another, depending on the milieu, pH, protein content, trace elements, heavy metals, etc. Humans live, therefore, in intensive symbiosis with a world of bacteria and micro-organisms which is also constantly changing according to the milieu, diet and the acid base condition of the person and is even developing endogenic proteins! So it is that bacteria in nature and in humans can change from one form into other forms and into stages of development and also constantly change their pathogenicity depending on the metabolic milieu. As a consequence, it is not necessary to assess bacteria, viruses and fungi as foreign to us but as a part of ourselves, and they can be altered in their pathogenity by correction of the inner milieu.

As a result, micro-organisms are not fixed units, they continually change. They arise – and this is what is special in pleomorphistic thinking – by upward development from endocellular components, which Enderlein named "protites" and Wilhelm Reich called "bions" but which nowadays are also called somatids and which are normally present in every human cell and every bodily fluid. Even more fascinating is the idea that these particles are given to us when we are created and later to a great extent "survive" us – that is, they go back to nature as a part of our self. They can withstand high temperatures up to 300°C, so they cannot be "killed off" by sterilisation. However, in a similar way they can also develop upwards from plant cells, as Wilhelm Reich proved when he grew bacteria and amoeba from sterile liquid from grass cells.

But Enderlein's most important finding was also the beginning of his effective isopathic therapy: the "high valencies" (i.e. the bacterial and fungal forms) can be reduced by the "low valencies" (i.e. the endogenic protites: proteins and nucleic acids) and developed upwards into non-pathogenic forms if these "low valencies" are present in sufficient number and the milieu is correct. So it becomes clear that the actual presence of these so-called "low valencies" and the correct cell and plasma milieu is very important for good immunity – that is, human beings acquire good resistance through the presence of the early stages of bacteria and viruses.

This is a completely new and dynamic way of looking at human integrity, demonstrating that it is the presence of an intensive exchange with the environment which is the basis of health and maturation. Bacteria and viruses are therefore not "harmful and dangerous and need to be wiped out", but their monomorphic design is only the expression of a rigid, blockade-induced, abnormal milieu. Antibiotics and similar remedies have thus become largely unnecessary, and even the monodiagnosis of fungi and bacteria loses its importance to a great extent.

Thus it becomes clear that the orthomolecular substances and acid base regulators previously referred to are a pre-requisite for successful isopathic therapy. They remove blockades which have arisen as a result of mineral deficits, hyperacidity or heavy metals and so permit the isopathic decomposition of the high valencies. However, the low valencies which arise as a result of isopathic therapy (protites, chondrites, symprotites) can again continue to exist in these forms only if the milieu of the environment suits them; for this vitamins, minerals and Alkala N are necessary, and that is another reason why we use them.

Darkfield microscopy of the native blood is a very suitable method of assessing vitality and the pleomorphic dynamics of the blood. In this type of assessment one drop of vital blood is taken using a capillary tube and observed in the native state in the darkfield under 1200 times magnification. The dynamic change of the structures is observed over a period of time, and this gives an insight into the tendency of the cells to degenerate and into the endobiontic contamination of the plasma. In this investigation the following questions can be answered from the dynamics:

- Milieu

- Excess of acid / excess of protein

- Toxic or other blockades

- Activity of the leucocytes: that is, contamination / toxicity of the leucocytes

- Endobiontic contamination

- Evidence of the therapeutic approaches which are necessary

- Acid base therapy / isopathic therapy / immune stimulation

- Detoxification therapy needed / diet therapy needed.

Darkfield diagnosis of the native blood is the only test which at the same time shows us the milieu and the degenerative tendency of cellular elements as well as the buffering load on the blood. It is suitable, particularly when observed over a period of several hours, for demonstrating stress loads on the blood cells and thus tendencies to develop certain diseases, even pointing to tendencies to develop tumours. In addition, conclusions about diseased organs and even about archetypal psychological themes can be drawn analogously by interpretation of the blood crystals and the protein condensates in the blood. The method is very important for patients with tumours for assessing their ability to tolerate chemotherapy.

No other test shows the relationship between the patient's condition and Reckeweg's phases of illness as clearly as darkfield microscopy can. And every darkfield constellation has its own related biological and milieu therapy. Darkfield microscopy is therefore a test which is very quick, very practical and very motivating for the patient.

The isopathic remedies, manufactured by reductions from high valencies, are (according to Enderlein) the core products for therapy. They lead to a fundamental re-tuning of the "inner milieu", of the bacterial world and the protein milieu, but must also be selected to suit the patient's constitution and prescribed over a long period of time. To increase their effectiveness, the main remedies in this range (Nigersan, made from *Aspergillus niger*, and Mucokehl, made from Mucor racemosus) should be combined intermittently with the homeopathic metabolic products of this same fungal stage, namely Acidum lacticum (Sanuvis) and Acidum citricum (Citrokehl). The products in this range are: Mucokehl, Nigersan, Notakehl, Fortakehl, Mucedokehl, Pefrakehl, Albicansan, Larifikehl, Pinikehl, Quentakehl, and the combination remedies Exmykehl and Sankombi.

The **immune biological products** stimulate the bacteria and lead to stimulation of the macrophages and also of the lymph cells, in particular the T-cells, which is scientifically well-substantiated, so that with the range of Sanum therapies it is possible to bring about active macrocytal resorption and immune fixing of pathological proteins. Depending on the choice of immune biologicals (bacterial remedies), either T-cell activity, particularly in viral illnesses, can be stimulated (e.g. *Propionibacterium avidum* or *Mycobacterium phlei*) or stimulation can be given by activating and fixing macrophages (e.g. with Recarcin) against the long acting forms of bacteria which are becoming more and more common. Immune modulation using the immune biological remedies is particularly effective in cases of chronic dysbiosis (bacterial "nests" in the crypts of the bowel) and also particularly in cases where there is siphonospores as an inevitable result of dead teeth (Arthrokehlan/ corynebacterial remedies). And of course in cases of holistic medicine and above all in the treatment of dental foci of interference one should not forget the immune biological remedy Arthrokehlan A. Remedies in this group: Utilin, Utilin "S", Latensin, Recarcin, Arthrokehlan A and U, Propionibacterium avidum, Bovisan.

Finally the range of haptens (Sanukehl's) rounds off milieu therapy as the absolutely targeted regulation therapy: the low-molecular polysaccharides have the ability to bond antigens and to improve their identification by macrophages; they therefore intervene in auto-immune processes and tumours. The antigenicity of the proteins is in these cases desirable, and the haptens increase it in such a way that the previously blockaded immune system is once again "started up".

This mechanism is particularly important in diseases where there are tumours, where there is hardly any antigenicity remaining in the tumour cells, and in cases after treatment with antibiotics. After the bacteria have been destroyed with antibiotics, the latter do not have the same antigenicity as the remnants of the cell walls and the bacteria, and therefore they are no longer recognised by the macrocytal immune system, which can lead to so-called "auto-immune" diseases. The haptens mark these "part antigens" and convert them into more recognisable antigens, so that a normal immune reaction becomes possible again. Milieu therapy which is properly understood can thus lead to a very clear improvement in the body's ability to react and first gives the body the ability to react to energetic methods.

Milieu therapy therefore is the best possible supplement for all types of energetic therapy and is often the pre-requisite for preparing a patient before treatment with homeopathy or fine energy.

The connection between the teeth and the inner milieu

Milieu therapy is an essential precondition for every biological therapy, just like **thorough cleaning of the teeth**, as the blockading toxins come from diseased teeth: siphonospores as long-acting bacteria which have a bacterial toxic and probably very carcinogenic effect on the mesenchyme, but also have a highly toxic effect as a result of deadly proteins (thioethers, mercaptans, indols). American researchers (Weston

Price et al.) were able to show that in every dead tooth in the dentine canal – i.e. in the organic substance - there are inevitably siphonospores which are also found in large quantities in tumour tissues. These lead to decay of the pulp structures as in a corpse and thus produce amounts measured in nanogrammes of already antigenic and highly toxic bodily poisons, which on the one hand are washed out over the mesenchyme and on the other hand also generate a high level of interference on the meridian, which is probably why dead teeth (all teeth which have been subjected to root treatment are dead and ridden with siphonospores!) tend to interfere first with their meridian processes. Every tooth is linked to a meridian; that is, every meridian has its own specific groups of teeth.

It is interesting that for example in periodontitis for the most part either the dead teeth or the tooth groups of a corresponding meridian are periodontal, and therefore the tooth can give the doctor very valuable pointers to the meridian which is affected by interference. Periodontitis therefore almost always includes interference with the meridians and problems with the milieu and must also be treated correspondingly.

However, the teeth are also the sources of contamination by heavy metals, in particular mercury. The doctor should also always consider palladium, tin and aluminium which can cause similar high-grade contamination of the cells. According to Enderlein these heavy metals are also typically the cause of the blockades ("Mochlosen") which reduce the vital upward and downward development of the endobiontic valencies (see above) and therefore fundamentally hinder the adaptation and regulation of cells and tissues, thus also being the true cause of bacterial or viral monoinfections. Likewise "Mochlosen" can come about as a result of electromagnetic and geopathic stress, fixed hyperacidity, and also a degenerative constitution. This again explains why people under stress of this type are more susceptible to bacterial and viral illnesses, as their dynamic system of downward and upward development of viruses and bacteria does not function.

The **excretion remedies for heavy metals** are Seleno-methionine, Selenokehl, Zinkokehl, Alkala N, Okoubasan, Cerivikehl, but also Pleo Chelate (a remedy from the chelates group) and ionic exchangers. The release of heavy metals from the teeth and their fixation to the target organs – ganglions, nerve cells and fibrocytes – are very dependent on the type of constitution as well as on the tissue content of antagonists and on the level of acid in the tissues. Again, this level can be influenced easily and effectively with the Sanum milieu remedies (foundation remedies, minerals).

The **biological milieu therapy** described in this article must be continued over a long period of time – that is, from several months to two years – and be accompanied by a healthy diet low in animal protein. It can lead to a fundamental regeneration of the tissues even in old people and to the healing of even long-term illnesses, and also to a harmonious extension of consciousness for the person. It is particularly suitable in cases of susceptibility to infection, chronic bacterial diseases, all diseases of the circulation and heart. It is also the foundation therapy for diseases involving tumours.

Dr. Thomas Rau, M.D.
Paracelsus Klinik Lustmühle,
9062 Lustmühle (bei St.Gallen)
Switzerland

Published in Sanum Post No. 46 1999
Copyright © 1999 Dr. Thomas Rau
All Rights Reserved

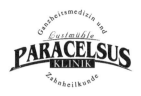

5

Professor Enderlein's Isopathy and Milieu Therapy – What is it?

The German microbiologist, physician and researcher, Prof. Dr. Günther Enderlein, was able to prove in his studies that microorganisms in the human body can develop upward from apathogenic forms via physiological early phases into pathogenic agents. In his research, he looked at fresh blood under a darkfield microscope. He demonstrated that it was exclusively the patient's *milieu interieur* (internal environment) that was responsible for the formation of viral, degenerative and even bacterial diseases. Modifying this milieu in the direction of physiological conditions is thus the way to counter most infectious and bacterial diseases. The milieu is determined by the **acid-base balance**, by the organism's **protein count** – in particular excess animal protein, which cannot be integrated into the body's cells – by the amount of **trace elements**.

Hyperacidity of the organism (tissue hyperacidity) is the result of long-term poor nutrition, usually over-rich in protein, but also an increasing lack of trace elements and minerals (chromium, selenium, magnesium, calcium) with alkalinizing effects. By means of a proper diet, plus supplying the missing trace elements, base equivalents and isopathically effective medications, the internal milieu an be improved to such a degree that chronic diseases can be influenced and their development reversed.

The Theory of Isopathy and the use of isopathic remedies, made from fungi, give us an easy to use and very effective instrument for the treatment of acute and chronic diseases. Prof. Dr. Enderlein's great achievement is having systemized the knowledge of the structures

(Endobionts) which colonise man. When they are of low-valence and physiologically developed, they are vital to many metabolic processes, particularly to materials transport in and out of the cells, as well as to blood coagulation. If these structures become of a higher-valence as a result of unphysiological milieu changes, they can cause various bacterial diseases – or, if general regulatory processes become blocked, viral diseases. He was able to demonstrate beyond a shadow of doubt that these developmental cycles which evolve pathological structures and germs all run similar courses. Professor Enderlein was able to demonstrate the three major developmental cycles, which respectively produce, in their culminant stages, the fungus *Mucor racemosus fresen, Aspergillus niger* and *Penicillium notatum.*

In each of these developmental chains (Cyclogenies) one finds certain bacteria and thus certain diseases or syndromes. Thus, the precursor stages of *Mucor racemosus* typically develop endothelial and endodermal diseases, and diseases of the circulatory systems. The diseases of the *Aspergillus niger* cycle, on the other hand, primarily affect connective tissue and ectodermal organs and therefore give rise to diseases of the tuberculin type, degenerative diseases and diseases of the connective tissue organs. Finally, *Pencillium notatum* exhibits in its precursor stages the agents of acute putrefying infections, staphylococci and streptococci, and the patients thus tend to acute bacterial illnesses and kidney/bladder disorders.

Professor Enderlein made the interesting discovery that diseases of the corresponding Cyclogenies could be treated to excellent result with the physiological early stages (low valences) of the corresponding cycles. The isopathic remedies therefore contain the physiological and high-energy early structures, obtained via ultra-filtration, from the *Mucor racemosus, Aspergillus niger, Penicillium notatum* or Candida cyclodes.

Darkfield Microscopy

Using this microscopic investigation of fresh blood, the milieu, cell material exchange, a patient's degenerative tendency and the protein situation can all be evaluated. One can quickly get an idea of which therapies are needed-for example whether immune system stimulation or isopathic therapy should come first.

Darkfield microscopy is a very quick and clinical-practice-friendly method for evaluating the acid-base balance, excess protein and also **Endobiontic stress**. The determination of the degree of severity of a "blood mycosis" is thus possible and even practical in the day-to-day general practice.

Enderlein's teachings and his therapy make it possible to enable access to topics such as Candida and blood mycoses, but also to degenerative tendency and cancer susceptibility. In addition, cross-connections to other areas of holistic medicine such as homeopathy or Chinese medicine are made more understandable.

Dr. Thomas Rau, M.D.
Paracelsus Klinik Lustmühle,
9062 Lustmühle (bei St.Gallen)
Switzerland

Published in Explore! Volume 7 Number 1, 1996
Copyright © 1996 Dr. Thomas Rau
All Rights Reserved

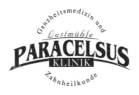

6

Thoughts on the Changeability of Microbes. Pleomorphism, Isopathy and Modern Research into Prions.

The research into the structure of prions has taken another step forward; we have gone further into the details of what are supposed to be Nature's wrong tracks. It is a matter of finding the one substance, which bonds with prions and neutralises their effect. Does it actually cause "mad cow disease" and the terrible Creutzfeldt-Jakob syndrome in humans, as is generally supposed nowadays? It is now believed that we can get closer to finding these substances if we could change their structure, with the result that when treating a patient it would not be possible to give microbial particles to drive out the former prions.

For us, this research – however strong the determination and enthusiasm of our scientists – is an example of narrow vision and a loss of regulative, functional thinking in medicine such as has been practised in cancer research for many years now. Research is being carried out into small details, instead of an attempt being made to recognise the significance of a development which leads to the fact that the body creates within itself components which can destroy it. It is a question of fighting the causes, not the effect. So we see parallels with cancer treatment and research, which for years also misguidedly resulted in no practical results or new forms of treatment. In research we are taking too little account of the basic problem, that is, the disruption to the dynamics of the living organism, just as little as in orthodox treatments. It is not being borne in mind that a human being is a part of the whole, of the earth in its completeness, and therefore it must of necessity also contain in itself rhythms of growth (of "self-destruction") in analogy to all living creatures on the earth.

The fundamental principles of organic life

Every living organism is an adaptive, dynamic system which can only maintain its inner balance if it keeps a constant eye on the changing environmental conditions. In holistic medicine we call this "regulation". Regulation is an expression of reactivity, vitality and also of an intact whole-body system. The fundamental principle of regulation is phylogenetic development, the development which our genes have made over thousands of years. We call this fundamental "understanding" of the body as to how it has to adapt "information", and we know that it is stored not only in genetic material but also in the proteins and intercellular material where the immune cells can also be found.

The great German researcher Professor Günther Enderlein proved back in the years before the war that the smallest protein corpuscles, of which every mammal and human being has huge numbers, are already present at their procreation in ovum and sperm and are therefore passed on by parents at birth, but they can also be acquired later from external sources and live in us for the whole of our life. These protein corpuscles known as "protites" and the conglomerate forms of them which are present in every cell and bodily fluid of warm-blooded creatures known as "symprotites" are low-molecule protein chains of a few hundred amino acids – that is, "organic peptides" – and their stearic structures link with each other in a spiral shape and are characterised by the sequence of amino acids and the S- or N-atoms binding them together. Protites must therefore have a molecular weight of about 7,000 to 10,000, which also explains the fact that they are commonly found in the kidneys.

Very interesting connections have been shown in a new piece of research by Ch. Germer (Vienna 1996/97). Using 2D electrophoresis, Germer was able to show that in biochemical terms the main part of the "darkfield corpuscle" (symprotite) matched the protein structure of globin from the erythrocytes, and this points to the close connection between endobiosis and cell respiration. As a result, endobionts move into a position where their significance for the origin of every form of aerobic life becomes clear.

When these proteins accumulate, they become spherical structures which are colourless, heat resistant and insoluble (Heinz corpuscles), which is exactly how they are to be found in tumour cells. These research results also show that Enderlein was right in saying that endobionts in cancer cells are to be found in upward-developing high valencies or have an effect on the degeneration of the cell.

These "symbionts" can be acquired from external sources almost only through cellular material of animal origin, such as in foodstuffs. Here again, the way animals are kept and thus their inner milieu determines the virulence of these proteins acquired from external sources. In this way human beings are already intensively caught up in and linked into the relationships within nature.

Years ago a researcher who actually worked with Enderlein, Dr Wolfram Seyfarth MD, pointed to these relationships and demonstrated that the mitochondria in our cells have the potential to develop their own "in-house" bacteria and that where other micro-organisms can develop as a result of the decomposition of bacteria, viruses can also develop. This also explains why treatment with antibiotics in the long term favours the development of viral pathogens, as the bacterial products of the decomposition of the cells are the fundamental structure on which microbes can develop. Professor Enderlein also proved that in unfavourable conditions these symbionts can become lumpy , develop in an upward direction and become very virulent, developing upwards into viruses, bacteria and (in a strong shift of the milieu) even into fungi. Interestingly, Enderlein also described how nucleic acid (DNA) develops from the protein particles of the protites during their upward development, this too being a carrier of information and genetic material. This finding can be regarded as a significant impulse for a change of paradigm in medicine and biology.

As everybody knows, Enderlein and the researchers working with him described constant microbial as "pleomorphism" – that is, the science of change. We also see similar approaches in the very old, tried and tested teachings of Ayurvedic and Chinese medicine, only with complete different ideas. Enderlein called these protein particles "protites" and observed that in cell metabolism these take on functions which are important for life, such as maintaining the viscosity of the cells and bodily fluids and the transport of materials. But he also found that they can multiply in number between the cells, become lumpy and change until the host cell is destroyed, according to the milieu present.

Particularly where there are obstruction factors, the ability to change can be blocked and expressed in the phase of an isolated single microbe. It is then no longer possible for the pathogenic high valencies to regress endogenically. Enderlein called this "mochlosis" (the Greek for a "state of obstruction") and demonstrated that this happens predominantly where there is contamination by electromagnetism, a lack of trace elements and toxic foci, but particularly in cases of heavy metal contamination. Enderlein and also his later co-worker Dr Baum discovered these connections as they were incubating blood cultures from humans and animals and found that bacterium cultures and even fungal cultures were developing. But if they added heavy metals to these blood samples, or if they changed their acid-base milieu or the protein content, only certain monocultures formed which then no longer changed themselves dynamically, i.e. they were "blocked". This also explains the fact that in human beings whose milieu is contaminated by heavy metals, bacterial and viral problems developed at an increasing rate. Isn't it true that we nowadays see these very factors widespread in monocultures, in manured ground, in soil which is contaminated with toxins, the products of which our cattle eat and concentrate? Also in the massive electromagnetic contamination to which we and our animals are subjected by short wave transmitters, radio telephones, etc?

The dangers of treatment with antibiotics
If you imagine that pathogens in the body arise as a result of the agglomeration of proteins which thereby change their character, then it is also clear that treatment with antibiotics cannot be successful in the long term. By using them we only destroy the bacteria, opening up their membranes, but fragments remain in the body from which microbes can again grow, according to the pathological milieu remaining. But the opening up of bacteria using antibiotics, particularly in the case of fungi, can even release highly poisonous bacterial toxins which are able to

interfere with the cells and nerve functions. Contrary to this, milieu therapy according to Enderlein makes the milieu unsuitable for them and therefore turns them back into normal non-pathogenic protites.

In his time Professor Enderlein did not receive any recognition for this work, as this particular piece of knowledge regarding the dynamic development of viruses, bacteria and fungi in the organism and in human cells was considered unthinkable, as was the fact that a protein (not DNA!) can alter the genes of a human being. We find it wonderful that, as a result of the new research being carried out, Professor Enderlein's view is being justified. The person who really discovered the "prion" is Professor Enderlein. He was the first to describe how the proteins from which microbes come appear in every human being in physiological form but change to a pathogenic form mainly as a result of the wrong diet, just as the PrP proteins of the prion are altered cell proteins from every cell of the body. The cause of this mal-development is the giving of feed made from dead bodies to other animals – a grotesque form of faulty diet for naturally totally vegetarian cattle and sheep which goes back over many generations of animals.

But Professor Enderlein made other discoveries which are even more important: every upward development of the protites (= symbionts) is strictly dependant on the inner milieu, the trace element content, the electromagnetic and redox potential of the cells, and above all the diet. Shouldn't we make a start here, in other words carry out research into the influence of long-term change of the inner milieu, which is the real cause of chronic diseases?

An example: cattle which developed the BSE virus had been fed on "super-feed" containing ingredients of animal origin. In fact, the leftovers from slaughterhouses had been given to the cattle in the form of meat and bonemeal which of course still contained the aforementioned animal, mal-developed protite forms. But Professor Enderlein demonstrated that temperatures above boiling point do not alter the protites (prions) at all, that they can even withstand temperatures up to 340 degrees as well as deep freezing and drying for thousands of years. He proved this by examining the dust in Egyptian pyramids which had come from mummies, where the aspergillus fungus protites were still active, had even achieved very high valencies as a result of the mummification treatment and were capable of causing very severe lung diseases among the archaeologists.

The prospects of holistic milieu therapy

We see, therefore, that the inner milieu makes the most important contribution to the healing of chronic viral diseases. Bonding or neutralising the BSE prion will have no permanent effect, for a basic principle of nature underlies this, namely the maintenance and protection of species. New viruses and particles which will make us ill will keep on appearing so long as we do not support and build up the inner parts (cell milieu, fluid milieu) of our cattle and animals but also of human beings by keeping them correctly and making sure that they have the right sort of lifestyle and diet. It has already been shown in the case of hepatitis (viral disease), AIDS and other viral diseases that new forms are continually appearing and that there is no point in targeting them specifically as this does not attack the reason for their development. However, if we change the lifestyle, the diet and in particular the othomolecular milieu of the person, then no further viral disease develops or it becomes so weak as to be of no significance.

The othomolecular milieu of human beings (trace element, vitamin and mineral content) can easily be determined using biological medical tests: hair mineral analysis, darkfield microscopy of the vital blood, heavy metal levels in the urine, etc. In this way we see that people with recurrent viral infections can improve their ability to regulate quite significantly through such treatment and after a few months do not suffer any more relapses. Even chronic viral diseases like herpes, neuralgia and even hepatitis disappear as the body can now cope by itself with the now smaller number of virulent particles.

Professor Enderlein also discovered that the "high valencies" (that is, the "agglomerated" large forms of the protites) can be reduced and destroyed by their apathogenic low valencies. This is the basic idea behind isopatic therapy or "isopathy": that is, therapy using endogenic substances. The SANUM-Kehlbeck isopathic remedies used in this type of treatment contain the apathogenic low valencies for the majority of important "disease" pathogens. The best-known of these medications are the remedies MUCOKEHL and NIGERSAN, made from the fungus cultures of Mucor racemosus and the mould Aspergillus niger. The combination of this form of therapy with the orthomolecular therapy and change of diet described above brings about quite striking results in the treatment of chronic viral diseases and infections. This truly biological therapy also has a real effect on most immunisations – in particular hepatitis, which we cannot recommend, or influenza immunisations.

The consequences of the knowledge which we have acquired

- Grazing animals should not be given any feed of animal origin at all during their lifetime, in order to stop the spiral of "upward development". Calves should not be fed with milk from mother cows which themselves have given feed containing ingredients of animal origin.

- For as long as this cannot be guaranteed, meat from grazing animals should not be eaten.

- The consumption of meat by humans and the consumption of milk (milk contains the same protites and high valencies) should be restricted to the minimum. We recommend a vegetarian diet, or at the most a meat meal once or twice a week of poultry which has been raised without hormones or feed containing meat and bonemeal.

- Strict attention must be paid to the replacement of minerals in cereal fields and vegetable fields. Particular attention should be paid to selenium, manganese and magnesium and these should be given as a supplement in organic form.

- In patients with chronic illnesses, viruses and infections the first line of approach is treatment of the inner milieu with alkaline therapy, diet, trace elements, best based on an analysis of the individual 's requirements using the investigations mentioned above.

- More time and effort in medical research should be devoted to the subjects of the milieu, orthomolecular connections and acid-base balance.

The interesting opportunities of low valencies which have proved of great practical benefit in our work should be more thoroughly researched.

Professor Enderlein's research should be reproduced using modern methods and taken up by our young, active researchers with the enthusiasm it deserves.

Dr. Thomas Rau, M.D.
Paracelsus Klinik Lustmühle,
9062 Lustmühle (bei St.Gallen)
Switzerland

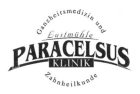

7

Allergies, What now?
Causes, Clarification and Holistic Treatment of Allergies

Causes of Allergies from the Holistic Point of View

Allergies are over-reactions of the immune system. The immune system is (from the holistic point of view) an extremely complex system, comprising the white blood system (lymphocytes, granulocytes, macrophages, mast cells), as well as the entire system of mucous membranes. It also is closely involved with the normally present bacterial colonies in the mucous membranes.

An allergy is therefore not just an overreaction to an allergen (trigger substance); sensitivity to an allergen is merely the very tip of the iceberg. Only an organism with a severely disturbed internal milieu reacts allergically. To be sure, the internal milieu disturbance is usually not noticed, since it is chronic and tends to build up gradually over time. However, treatment (see below) must always be oriented to this basis, i.e. the internal milieu.

Allergens. Allergies can be caused by the most varied of substances and materials, e.g. cat hairs, hay dust, strawberries, etc. All allergies which can be determined by the use of skin tests are secondary allergies, which only appear because of underlying basic allergies (usually foodstuffs, see below) and severely damaged mucous membranes and a seriously disturbed internal milieu.

Avoiding the secondary allergens – i.e. the putative trigger substances – therefore only gives temporary relief. Thus, it makes no sense to embark on major environmental alteration campaigns, such as thorough house-cleaning for presumed allergy to dust, since much greater success can be attained by eliminating the additional trigger factors (see the diagram of the six-pillar model of allergies in the first paper On the Nature of Biological Medicine). The basic allergen, as described below, is usually to be found among the basic components of one's diet, those served from early childhood – usually cow's milk, nuts and eggs. Thus, most allergies are the consequences of a dietary protein sensitivity, which, for its part, is not directly noticed.

Hyperacidity. As described in earlier papers, hyperacidity (usually diet-based) affects the organism's entire regulatory ability. Mast cells (which trigger allergic reactions upon coming in contact with allergens) de-granulate much more easily in an acidic milieu and are more likely to generate histamines. Therefore, one of the most important steps in allergy therapy is generating an alkaline milieu in the organism. De-acidification of the organism must be done consistently for 1-2 years, by means of dietary redirection (little or no animal protein, few milk products and no sugar) and the use of alkaline powders such as Alkala N.

Dysbiosis (intestinal mucous membrane changes and defective intestinal flora). The intestinal flora, comprising some billions of bacteria, form a fine film on the inside of the intestinal tube. Everything man eats must pass through this bacterial lawn, which alters and filters the foodstuffs. This bacterial colonization has grown up along with man, and has, in its symbiosis, fully adapted itself to the interests of the organism as a whole. When the intestinal flora are not intact, e.g. due to treatment with antibiotics, or ingestion of food which has itself been treated with antibiotics, or heavy metals, then the intestinal mucous membrane's absorptive abilities become impaired.

Then, proteins are absorbed wrongly, so that they cannot wholly be broken down. The villi then become less dense, and foreign proteins can then penetrate the intestinal mucous membrane. These are detected by the immune system, which then reacts accordingly. Over 80% of the human immune system is thus situated alongside the intestines. It is therefore understandable that disturbances of the intestines and the intestinal flora place a tremendous overload on the immune system, which then often reacts "allergically" to otherwise quite innocuous proteins. Allergies are thus usually indirect ailments of the intestinal mucous membrane. Thus, in treating allergy patients, the greatest attention needs to be given to restoring the intestinal flora and the intestinal mucous membrane. The intestinal flora are restored with a vegetarian diet high in raw vegetables, and by avoiding animal protein (including dairy products).

Toxins/Heavy Metals/Mercury. There is a direct relationship between frequency of exposure to mercury and frequency of allergic ailments. Heavy metals block the functions of the lymphocytes and macrophages and thus block man's defensive systems. This can be seen most impressively in a darkfield investigation of vital blood.

Mercury can be transferred to infants from amalgam fillings in the mothers' teeth. Later on, environmental pollution (lead and aluminum) and one's own amalgam fillings massively elevate the toxic burden. Therefore, in treating allergies, one must always look for mercury poisoning (DMPS Test) and the corresponding diversion (detoxification) must be carried out. The Paracelsus Klinik Lustmühle, working together with its dental division, and based on its many years of experience, has worked out a detailed system for mercury detoxification. This, has shown striking success in treating patients with neurodermitis, asthma and juvenile allergies.

Heavy metal toxicity is becoming ever more common and can usually be detected with a hair mineral analysis, especially aluminum and lead. Mercury poisoning cannot be detected in this manner, since mercury "infests" connective tissue and nerves and migrates to the skin only to a very slight degree.

Vitamins and trace elements, e.g. selenium, zinc, manganese, Vitamins E and C, are used to treat and bind/eliminate heavy metals. The chelating agents Dimaval (DMPS) or EDTA can also be used to bind mercury. This is an extremely effective heavy-metal detoxification therapy – which, however, must be done under a physician's supervision and guidance, because it can lead to mineral and trace element deficiencies. The chelate infusions we perform have enormous success in detoxification.

Fungi. A nearly mandatory part of the multicausal (i.e. an illness that has multiple causes) nature of allergies is fungal infestation. Proving systemic mycosis (usually *Aspergillus niger* or Candida) is difficult, which is why orthodox medicine very often casts doubt on a fungal presence. The patients exhibit – besides the typical allergy – other signs such as fatigue, susceptibility to infection, frequent bladder or vaginal inflammations, lack of concentration, depression, eye disorders, dizziness and other neurological disorders. Antibody and skin tests are usually negative and yet the patients feel quite ill; they are then often written off as psychosomatic cases. A darkfield microscopic examination of vital blood exposes the "fungification" with the characteristic alterations of the blood cells and the plasma.

Darkfield microscopy thus represents an excellent investigative method for evaluating the acid-base milieu, hyperproteinemia, the blood's degenerative tendency and evaluation of a possible "fungification". Therefore, any treatment of allergies must include a concomitant treatment of the blood milieu with homeopathic/isopathic products from the fungal line (Professor Enderlein's isopathic therapy).

With this combined treatment using isopathic fungal preparations, treatment of the hyperacidity and detoxification, practically any allergy can be markedly improved, given time, as long as the primary allergens in the diet (usually cow's milk, eggs and nuts) are also strictly avoided.

Avoiding the allergen is often not feasible (for example, in spring, it is difficult for a person with pollen allergy to avoid pollen; people with so-called "house-dust" allergies can hardly avoid some contact with their allergen). However, with the above described treatment, this is not so necessary – so that, although we advise the beleaguered allergy patient to avoid the allergen, it is usually not really necessary because of the above treatment.

The described allergy therapy lasts for about 1-2 years, and must be carried out without interruption. However, the patients are then well and truly healed, which – especially for severe allergic diseases such as asthma, neurodermitis, rheumatic disorders or candida infestation – motivates the patients to do their part.

Histamines – The histamine supply comes almost exclusively via the diet – animal proteins, fish, shellfish (but also tomatoes) are very rich in histamines. Avoiding animal proteins, especially pork, venison, fish and eggs is therefore very important for allergy sufferers.

Primary Allergens
As described above, the primary allergens usually go unnoticed, and the dietary allergy nearly always expresses itself by means of other symptoms.

Symptoms of Dietary Allergy in Infants, Children and Adults
A primary allergy to dietary elements usually develops during infancy, when the infant is fed foreign animal protein which its intestinal mucous membrane system cannot yet process. Bovine milk proteins, for example, are thus taken into the body in an insufficiently processed form, where they function as foreign protein allergens and induce an immune response in the Peyer's Patches of the immune system, which lie alongside the intestines. If cow's milk is then later ingested, the organism reacts with a continuous immune response, which can lead to exhaustion of the immune system and the characteristic susceptibility to infection and other sequelae.

It is therefore of utmost importance not to give infants, up to an age of about 12 months, any dairy products, eggs or nuts, which all function as allergens in infants. It is regrettable that most of the powdered baby formula mixes are made with cow's milk and thus represent, for predisposed children, a high allergen risk. Therefore, children up to the age of 1 year should only be given mother's milk or soy-substitute formulas.

The Significance of Infestation by Molds and Candida
The significance of mold infestation (*Aspergillus niger* and *Mucor racemosus* and their respective predecessor stages) has been described above. Most allergy patients also suffer from mold infestation. Unfortunately, orthodox medicine does not yet recognize this fact, although it turns up nearly every time under subtle energy testing. The presence of this infestation is also explained by the patient's impaired metabolic milieu – so common among allergy sufferers – which provides

a very favorable environment for the upward development of the fungal stages. Thus, in advanced cases, antibodies to fungi and various allergens can frequently be found. The treatment (see below) must therefore always include measures against the organismic stress of fungal precursor stages.

Candida is a particularly current theme. Candida (yeast) is often named as the cause of allergic diseases or (in alternative-medicine circles) brought into close association with allergies. Candida colonization is often found in allergy patients, both through blood antibody determination as well as through stool cultures.

However, based on our own investigations, Candida is not the cause of the allergy, but rather the expression of a maladapted milieu – and also quite frequently of heavy-metal toxicity. Thus, a holistic allergy treatment quite often improves the Candida situation at the same time. On the other hand, an antimycotic/antibiotic candida treatment will do even more damage to the intestinal flora, thus further worsening the intestinal milieu and promoting allergic reactions even more.

Disturbance foci: Especially in allergic adults, disturbance foci are almost always found, the elimination of which can often improve allergic tendencies considerably.

Primary disturbance foci: Under certain circumstances, disturbance fields can trigger allergies. The commonest forms are:

- Dead and ingrown teeth, dental root granulomas, periodontosis

- Chronic tonsillitis (often with encapsulated pus foci), paranasal sinus inflammations

- Gallbladder diseases (with or without gallstones), chronic appendicitis

- Chronic inflammations in the region of the female sexual organs and – much less commonly – the male sexual organs

- Chronic small and large intestinal inflammations

- Scars of various kinds

Disturbance fields are chronic sub-symptomatic inflammations which exhibit remote action, partly by informational subtle energy means, partly via leukocyte activation. They affect the immune system by imposing a burden on the leukocyte/lymphocyte system.

Seeking out and eliminating disturbance foci can significantly improve the immune reaction, and thus the anti-allergic capability of the entire organism. The better the lymphocyte system reacts – including Peyer's Patches, the primary lymphocyte organs – the less the body needs to use the histamine/mast cell reaction as a defensive mechanism.

The main disturbance foci in children are, first, intestinal disorders and, second, chronically inflamed tonsils. However, these are usually compensation reactions following long-lasting overburdening of Peyer's Patches through poor nutrition in early infancy.

For adults, disturbance foci in the mandibular region (dead, root-treated and ingrown teeth, dental root granulomas) are the most common. Thorough holistic dental clarification, including the elimination of all dental disturbance foci – which usually includes extracting all dead teeth – is thus an important component of any allergy therapy.

Test methods
It is clear from the above that testing for specific allergens can only reveal the least part of the allergy problem and is thus seldom necessary. We frequently see patients come to us with long lists of alleged allergens, who have been tested by the most diverse methods. Yet, these are mostly secondary allergies, which lose their allergic ability when either the basic allergens of dietary proteins are avoided or the trace element and bacterial milieu is improved. It thus makes no sense to attempt desensitizatlon or "bio-resonance extinction" of individual allergens, whose effectiveness will be short-term at best.

For allergy testing, one must therefore investigate along a broader front:

- Skin tests for allergens: Most skin tests are not relevant, since they often yield false negatives and since the skin often exhibits reactions to substances which have no allergic significance for the organism as a whole. Besides which, the skin is, as an ectodermal tissue, a totally different reaction system than the mucous membranes, which usually generate the disturbing symptoms of allergies as part of their attempts at detoxification.

- Subtle energy testing: This includes electro-acupuncture, Biotensor, pendulums, Bioresonance testing, kinesic pulse testing (RAC) and kinesiology. All these tests are similar and all are based on the idea of the tester coming into resonance with the test subject. The tester must thus be highly sensitive, must be very good at maintaining a neutral state and must be able to register the vibrational changes of the test person. All of these tests have a highly subjective component, require a great deal of experience and are hardly ever reproducible, which means that they are not recognized by science and orthodox medicine. They do, however, have the advantage of high sensitivity and can thus be used as diagnostic hints. However, we always combine these methods with other test methods to arrive at a therapeutic indication.

It should also be kept in mind that subtle energy testing cannot be performed on many people, since they have masking disorders such as amalgam intoxication, dental foci or toxic blockages. For the same reason, these patients cannot usually be treated homeopathically; their blockades have to be broken up and detoxified first.

Professor Rost's Thermoregulation Diagnostics: This assessment – which is, unfortunately, practised at only a very few places in Switzerland – focuses on the patient's diet and the resultant disturbance of the intestinal milieu, but also of the lymphatic system. However, this cannot indicate the primary allergen, but merely the allergic hyper-regulatory reaction to it. Nevertheless, this test is very important to us in allergy clarification, since with it the question of foodstuff allergy can be settled – and the same test can also determine disturbance foci in the organism, such as old blockages and foci in the paranasal sinus region, tonsil region or the lower body (for females), all of which are frequent causes of chronic ailments.

The disadvantage of Thermoregulation Diagnostics is the difficulty in evaluating the results, as well as the high price of the diagnostic apparatus.

Hair mineral analyses: This is a quite valuable test which returns results concerning trace elements, as well as heavy-metal toxicity. Allergy sufferers often exhibit low levels of zinc, selenium deficiency – but also high levels of phosphorus, magnesium and calcium (as a consequence of hyperacidity). High levels of aluminum are common in allergy patients. Lead and mercury toxicities block the white blood cells and thus impair immune reactions. Hair mineral tests are thus a good way to investigate the milieu.

Mercury tests: Mercury, originating in nearly all cases from amalgam fillings, can so alter the body's reactions as to trigger allergies. These are cases of mercury poisoning, which favors allergic reactions. Thus, we often can only heal neurodermatitis, skin eczemas, asthma and repeated maxillary sinusitis, as well as recurring bladder inflammations, by eliminating the mercury from the body of the patient.

Therefore, it is necessary to have a reliable mercury test method. At the Paracelsus Klinik Lustmühle, we use subtle energy testing and the Dimaval test. One needs direct material proof of mercury deposits in the body, and of the ability to eliminate them. If the values are elevated, then the mercury must always be eliminated from the body of the allergy patient – but the amalgam filling source must also be removed.

In the DMPS test, the overall mercury burden is evaluated – and also the patient's tendency to bind mercury (low initial value/higher second value = strongly binding and high total amount).

The heavy-metal urine test is a simple screening test which is based on color reactions to heavy metals. It has the advantage of yielding results simply and inexpensively, but gives no quantitative answers.

Darkfield investigation of vital blood: As mentioned above, this is a very valuable investigative method, yielding information on the body's milieu, the acid-base balance, infestation with fungal precursors, as well as information about toxic burdens of the leukocytes, i.e. reduction of immune ability.

All the above-named test methods make possible a broad-based and differentiated conclusion concerning the necessary therapies for allergy cases, which then in the vast majority of cases have a successful conclusion.

Hay fever, allergic asthma, food allergies, to some extent chronic skin allergies, can thus in most cases be cured with long-term therapy lasting 6 months to 2 years.

Treatment

Treatment has to consider all six of the Causal Pillars (see diagram in the paper on Biological Medicine): in acute treatment, the allergen must first be identified and avoided. In acute treatment, bioresonance with the Vegaselect device or Mora therapy often provides very good support. This energetic treatment "drowns out" (inverts) the allergen's information. But bioresonance therapy is never sufficient by itself, and is rather to be viewed only as a good adjunct measure. The most important thing is sticking to an anti-allergic (hypoallergenic) diet.

The hypoallergenic diet according to Werthmann and Rau:

- Total avoidance of cow's milk and all dairy products

- No pork, ham or bacon

- No eggs or egg products

- No food or drink which contains sugar

- No nuts of any kind

Most important is to avoid pork and dairy products. Cow's milk can be replaced by soya milk, goat or sheep milk, since these milks contains totally different proteins.

Isopathic Therapy

Isopathic fungal therapy using homeopathic/isopathic preparations can significantly alter the internal milieu of child patients: start with *Penicillium chrysogenum*, 10 drops 3 t.i.d. for 4 days, then change over to *Candida parapsilosis* and *Penicillium roquefortii*, 8 drops 2 t.i.d. for 7-

10 days, then finish, long-term, with *Mucor racemosus/Asperglllus niger* in combination 10 drops 2 t.i.d. for several months. In acute cases, e.g. hay fever, one can additionally administer *Aspergillus ruber* drops several times a day nasally and 8 drops 2 t.i.d. orally. All drops can be resorbed via the mouth and the nose. Salivate for a good long time and then swallow.

There also has to be an immunobiological build-up with trace elements, especially zinc, selenium, magnesium and manganese (Anti/Ox detox, Burgerstein firm) and with homeopathic/isopathic medications for stimulating the immune system: for children, *Bacillus subtilis* and *Bacillus firmus*, 2 drops rubbed into in the navel region or elbows daily for several months.

The lymphocyte system (Peyer's plaques) can be strengthened with the medication Peyer's patches extract, 1 capsule 2-3 t.i.d. for 2-6 months. Stimulation treatment with formic acid (Acidum formicium or potentised snake venom; for children, with catalysts of the citric acid cycle (Heel firm)).

Treating Susceptibility to Infection in Children

Susceptibility to infection in children is very often conditioned by a masked dietary allergy. Therefore, it is absolutely necessary to adhere to a low-allergen diet, especially for a few weeks or months at the beginning of therapy: no cow's milk or dairy products (since milk protein can have a highly allergenic effect), no pork, ham or bacon. Especially no sausages, hot dogs or cold cuts, since these are high in phosphates. No tropical fruits (citrus, etc.) and, initially, no eggs. In addition, the diet should be rich in minerals, i.e. lots of vegetables, eaten raw as much as possible. Sugar and sugar-containing food and drink to be avoided entirely (ice cream, candy bars, soft drinks, etc.).

Therapy

Initial therapy: *Penicillium chrysogenum*, 1-2 drops 3 t.i.d. nasal and 8 drops 3 t.i.d. oral. Hold in the mouth as long as possible, salivate, then swallow. Length of treatment: 1-2 vials.

After the *Penicillium chrysogenum, Mucor racemosus/Aspergillus niger* in combination, 8 drops 2 t.i.d. oral, salivate for a long time, then swallow. Length of this treatment: several months. In the case of acute infective relapse, start over again with *Penicillium chrysogenum* until the infection subsides, then *Mucor racemosus/Aspergillus niger* in combination again.

Peyer's patches extract capsules: take 1-2 capsules daily (for small children, open the capsule and sprinkle the powder in the mouth). Duration of this treatment: 2 packages. Afterwards, in the case of acute relapses or new infections begin again with 1 capsule 3 t.i.d.

Cleansing the lymphatic system: Lymphomyosot (Heel), 10 drops 3 t.i.d., important above all for children with swollen lymph nodes and tonsils.

To build up the immune system, after initial therapy, an immunobiological treatment is begun: *Bacillus subtilis* and *Bacillus firmus*, 2-3 drops rubbed into the elbows in daily alternation. After one vial, change over to *Mycobacterium phlei*, 1 capsule/week.

Taking Alen (a grain product very rich in minerals and vitamins) or multi-mineral tablets (Burgerstein) once a day is recommended, since the immune system and all cellular functions are very dependent on a good level of trace elements.

Dr. Thomas Rau, M.D.
Paracelsus Klinik Lustmühle,
9062 Lustmühle (bei St.Gallen)
Switzerland

Published in Explore! Volume 7 Number 2 1996

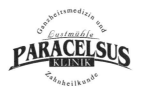

8

Susceptibility to Infection: Some Milieu and Isopathy-related Thoughts on a Frequent Topic

Excessive susceptibility to infection among children is one of the most common problems in general medical practice. At the Paracelsus Klinik – an outpatient clinic for Biological Medicine – this malady is registered in over 30% of treated juvenile patients. The definition of high juvenile infection susceptibility is: the child suffers more than 4 times a year from fever and at times painful inflammatory diseases with allergy symptoms, which many believe need to be treated with antibiotics. However, this is precisely the wrong approach, for the following reason: although the symptoms of the acute infective attack may be ameliorated more quickly, the ailment is never really cured, and in fact it is actually made worse. It is not the "naughty" bacteria that create the disease; rather these bacteria, which colonize every child and adult, are able to "be fruitful and multiply" because of a massively disturbed internal milieu.

The inner milieu (symbiontic bacterial world / acid-base condition of the tissues and bodily fluids / protein content / amount of foodstuff toxic residues) becomes disturbed when the patient's immune system and the child's nutrition are neglected over a long period of time. Usually the lymphatic system is disturbed, a situation which has become fixated and worked itself in since early childhood and which leads to immunological disturbances on into adulthood. Quite frequently, this disturbance is manifested by sensitivities/allergies to certain foods or intolerance to foodstuff ingredients. The connection between foodstuff sensitivities/allergies and infection susceptibility, as well as the lymphatic system, is as follows.

The Significance of the Intestinal/Lymphatic System for Man's Immunity

By far the greatest part of the substances that a person incorporates starting at birth is taken up via the intestinal tract. We thus have an enormous intestinal mucous membrane (in adults: 300 m² [nearly 1000 square feet]), which can absorb and process various substances. In order to be able to do this, the body needs an enormous number of intestinal bacteria (several trillion, which is more than the number of cells in the human body). These bacteria, first, prevent the colonization of the mucosa by disease-causing bacteria and, second, they create a fine film over the body's entire mucous membrane, upon which foreign substances are detected and foreign bacteria are killed off. These intestinal bacteria feed partly on cellulose from uncooked vegetables, which is why a high-vegetable diet is so important in building up the immune system.

The intestinal bacteria also partially cleave foreign proteins, thereby reducing their antigenic significance (cleaving the foreign proteins robs them of their allergy-inducing power).

The intestinal flora are thus the first barrier and the most important prerequisite for a functioning immune system. This is why it is so harmful to reach for antibiotics the moment the body is colonized by disease-triggering bacteria, since this also massively disrupts the intestinal flora and greatly reduces their numbers, since the antibiotics kill them as well.

Now, if foreign proteins that can disturb the immune system are taken up through the intestines (primarily animal proteins, which are recognized by the body as foreign and thus as allergens), then these are filtered out and processed by the immune system's second barrier, namely the Peyer's Patches (lymph nodes) situated along the inside intestinal walls. 80% of the human lymphatic and defensive system lies along the intestinal inner walls, in the form of minuscule lymph nodes. If these are overburdened over the long term by poor dietary habits, this leads over time to decompensation of the lymphatic system and thus the entire defensive system. The organism then reacts by trying to make up for poor lymph-node performance by creating many more lymph nodes, giving rise to the typical lymph-node and tonsil swelling (The adenoids and tonsils are clumps of lymph cells that only react when the intestinal immune system is overtaxed or decompensated).

Thus, the mucosa and lymph nodes of the facial/nasal region only react secondarily by swelling, constantly recurring inflammations and sensitivity. So, the more recourse is made to antibiotic treatment, the worse it is for the symbiontic bacterial defensive carpet and the patient's overall condition – which is why children then keep getting sick ever more frequently.

The Role of Cow's Milk in the Development of Infection Susceptibility

A very large segment of infection-susceptible children suffer from an allergy to cow's milk. This because cow's milk is the first foreign (nonself) protein the nursing infant is introduced to. These foreign proteins are administered to the poor infant in a baby bottle when there is not enough mothers' milk. But this milk protein cannot be cloven by the intestinal mucous membrane (still thin in early infancy), so that it is taken up nearly intact in its highly allergenic form and winds up in the lymphatic system beneath the mucous membrane. There, it is recognized as an allergen and the allergy lymph cells are trained to deal with this protein. These – in the sense of memory lymphocytes – then retain this orientation for the rest of the organism's life, thus laying the foundation for later food allergies. In the future, then, whenever cow's milk is ingested in whatever form, the lymphatic and immune systems are stimulated and, over the long term, overtaxed.

Treatment of infection susceptibility (see below) must therefore include lymphatic system therapy and a proper diet. Infection susceptibility is usually just the tip of the iceberg and never a disease in and of itself. It is always a matter of an immune system disorder, which can, however, express itself in various ways. As a result, the following symptoms occur:

Symptoms of Food Allergy in Infants and Children

- Increased susceptibility to infection
- Lymphatic system complaints (mucosal swelling/enlarged tonsils/repeated angina /restricted respiration)
- Milk crust (infantile eczema)
- Neurodermitis
- Chronic bloating, intestinal cramps
- Infantile colic

Symptoms in School-age Children and Adults

- Repeated infection, especially in the upper respiratory tract, ears, tonsils, paranasal/frontal sinuses
- Bronchial asthma
- Rheumatism
- Chronic fatigue
- Neurological disorders: hyperactivity, concentration disorders (school age)

How to Make Kids Stronger/Treating Infection Susceptibility

Thorough and consistent biological milieu therapy "reduces infection susceptibility and the recurring infections disappear within 1 to 2 years. The children who before were always ailing become the healthiest ones in their class. Those infections that still do occur (especially near the beginning of therapy) are lower in both intensity and frequency. They absolutely have to be treated biologically in order to avoid the backlash that antibiotic treatment brings. However, the decision on this therapy indication lies with the holistically oriented physician.

The treatment of infection susceptibility rests on four pillars.

1. Diet
2. Building up the intestinal flora and mucosa
3. Immune system build up
4. Elimination of toxins harmful to the intestinal tract and immune system

1. Diet

The infant's diet must consist exclusively of mother's milk. If this is not possible, then the infant must be nourished with soy milk at least until 12 months of age. Soy protein is significantly less allergenic and can be cloven by the mucosa even of small infants, and thus more easily taken up by the body. When fed soy milk formula, no deficiency whatsoever is created in the infant. Cow's milk is unsuitable for many children and should be strictly avoided for the first year, after which the infant's intestinal mucous membrane is able to cleave the allergenic cow-milk proteins. Most infant formula is made using cow's milk and therefore inadvisable. Giving the infant HA (hypoallergenic) formula is another possibility, but it is usually not necessary, and it is merely less (hypo-) allergenic, not completely allergy free.

Infants and school-age children with infection susceptibility need to avoid all contact with dairy products, as well as poultry protein, hen egg protein and white sugar. This includes all sweet drinks, milk products, especially yogurt. Also strictly prohibited are pork and pork sausages, and products with binding agents or preservatives that contain phosphates. The older infant's diet should be sure to include daily portions of raw vegetables, due to their high mineral content.

Forbidden:

- All cow's milk products
- Chicken eggs and egg products
- Nuts
- Citrus fruits (orange, mandarin, kiwi fruit, grapefruit)
- All food and drink containing white sugar
- No fruit in the evening due to fermentation

Recommended:

- All vegetables, potatoes, beans, rice and grain products
- All other fruits, eaten primarily morning and noon
- Soya products

2. Building up the intestinal flora and mucosa

Building up the intestinal system is done with bacterial products from Sanum, as well as by eating foods rich in cellulose, particularly finely grated raw vegetables (fennel, carrots, kohlrabi, etc.).

Building up intestinal flora: begin with Notakehl 3 x 8 drops daily for 7 days; repeat for every new disease attack. Next Pefrakehl 3 x 8 drops daily before meals, followed by Fortakehl 3 x 8 drops daily, each for about a week. After this initial treatment: Sankombi drops in nose and mouth, 3 x 8 drops in all, for 1-2 years.

3. Immune-system build-up with immunobiological medication

For small children, rub into elbow 2 drops daily Utilin N alternating with Recarcin N. For school-age children and adults, 1 capsule each of Utilin and Recarcin weekly (these are preparations made from bacteria, which are recognized as such by the immune system, but which cannot trigger disease and which builds up immunity).

For building up the Peyer's Plaques (lymphatic system along the intestinal inner walls): Rebas, initially 2 x 1 capsules for 10 days, and then 1 capsule daily. In acute cases, raise to 3 x 1 capsules for about a week.

4. Elimination of toxins harmful to the intestinal tract and immune system

All noxious and immune-taxing substances must be eliminated and, to counter them, a trace-element/multi-mineral therapy begun: multi-mineral/ vitamin tablets Cela (Burgerstein) 1-2 per day. All of these therapies must be kept up for 1-2 years. Mercury in amalgam fillings, lead and aluminium poisoning are quite common and can be detected (with a hair mineral analysis or a mercury elimination test (Dimaval test)) and treated accordingly by a biologically oriented physician. These immune-system weakening substances must absolutely be diverted. Infection-susceptible children must never undergo dental treatment involving metallic substances, particularly amalgam fillings.

Dr. Thomas Rau, M.D.
Paracelsus Klinik Lustmühle,
9062 Lustmühle (bei St.Gallen)
Switzerland

Published in Explore! Volume 7 Number 5 1996/97
Copyright © 1996 Dr. Thomas Rau
All Rights Reserved

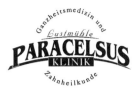

9

The Paracelsus Tumour Healthcare Programme

For over 10 years we have been carrying out intensive biological tumour therapy at the Paracelsus Clinic Lustmühle, up to now for outpatients and inpatients treatment. However, as a result of the incorporation of the Clinica Paracelsus Al Ronc we now have the opportunity to combine the experience gained over the past ten years with the advantages of intensive inpatient treatment with correct individual "cancer diet". The result is an intensive "Paracelsus Cancer Treatment Healthcare Programme" which provides a way into the biological & integrative treatment of malignant diseases and lays the "foundation" for follow-up treatment by your GP or specialist in biological therapies. The Paracelsus Tumour Healthcare Programme is unique and stands out particularly as a result of the combination of many different natural forms of therapy, some of which have already been very widely tested in "alternative" medicine and are already proven.

The Healthcare Programme is an extremely individual course of therapy, ideally lasting 3 weeks, which is suitable for patients with malignant diseases at any stage and is also very beneficial for patients who have already received or are still receiving orthodox treatment for their cancer.

We see the best results in the following tumours:

* prostate cancer / breast cancer in women

* metastatic forms of tumour of all types

- malignant tumours of the blood and lymphatic system (malignant lymphoma, chronic leukaemia, polycaethemia, thrombocytosis)

- cancer of the bladder (particularly in the interval between courses of therapy)

- tumours of the throat, pharynx and nasal regions

- colon and lung cancer (in combination or following orthodox treatments).

Our type of treatment is founded on a different way of looking at the development of the disease from that held by orthodox medicine. This is described below. Nevertheless, it is important that the patient should know that all doctors in the Paracelsus Clinics have undergone thorough training in orthodox medicine and also know a great deal about the various types of orthodox medical treatment for cancer.

Introduction and explanation:
The significance of degenerative and malignant diseases is both frighteningly high and increasing rapidly: their number and significance is beginning to far surpass those of other illnesses. In our grandparents' time only one person in about every ten or twelve was threatened by a malignant disease – in our day and age this has already risen to one person in three!

Although modern medicine has made undeniable progress in the area of acute illnesses, the treatment of malignant diseases poses almost insoluble problems for both doctors and patients. In many ways it would appear that cancers have taken over the position of the plagues of the Middle Ages; this applies particularly when you see the helplessness and perplexity which is frequently to be found among all concerned (including medical staff). This helplessness may be caused by the fact that people do not talk about the reasons why the cancer has occurred but simply try to treat the tumour.

Based on the findings of research carried out in the 19th century, the medicine of today is trying to tackle cancers using radical methods. At the present time these include surgery, radiation treatment and chemotherapy. In individual cases these are certainly sensible and even necessary (e.g. in the case of certain metastatic processes and in acute lymphoma and leukaemia), but in other cancers where observations have been made over a long period they have not helped (e.g. breast cancer in women, metastatic spread in the liver from tumours of the large intestine, prostate cancer).

In orthodox medical treatments it is regrettably often forgotten that the causes of cancer are many and varied and of an individual nature. The road to the point where cells degenerate and react against their human host is a long one. At the time when the diagnosis of cancer is made – if he/she is not given biological treatment and does not subsequently change his/her lifestyle – the patient has already gone nine-tenths of the way (or more!) along this road.

The low proportion of long-term successes and the often poor quality of life for people with cancer require that we change our way of thinking and take on board a complex combination of proven strategies from natural healing methods and regulatory medicine.

A few observations regarding the causes of cancer

In the biological treatment of cancer, the first priority is to treat the overloaded **ground system** (matrix or mesenchyme) of the cancer patient. This is the vital system of lymph, containing sugar and protein molecules which surrounds all the cells of the human body and through which all exchanges, cell nutrition and detoxification take place. Without the integrity of this system there can be no healthy and well-ordered cell growth. The wrong sort of diet or way of life, insufficient intake of essential substances, contamination with heavy metals and other toxins, as well as the chronic effect of so-called foci of interference (e.g. teeth which have been subjected to root canal treatment, scarred tonsils), result in loss of function of this important structure.

The intestines, immune system and cancer

It is necessary to stimulate the self-healing powers of the immune system which are always badly affected in cancer patients. This means in particular: activation of the so-called immunologically competent cells and restoration of the immunological vigour of the intestinal immune system.

Tests carried out in the past few years prove that people with cancer always have inadequate detoxification functions and serious changes in the intestine and/or immune system. The intestine is the most important immune organ in that its walls are home to approx. 80% of all lymph cells and the intestinal bacteria which are capable of rapid regeneration have important detoxification functions. Therefore: there should be no biological cancer therapy without a change of diet and bowel treatment!

Antioxidants, trace elements and vitamins

Minerals, vitamins and trace elements are regenerative and protect the tissues and may even inhibit cancer cells. Today everage nutrition and environmental influences considerably hinder the uptake of these. The Paracelsus Tumour Healthcare Programme integrates diagnosis on the basis of individual need and treatment with these substances, which is known as **orthomolecular medicine.**

Contamination with heavy metals

Heavy metals and toxic substances are carcinogenic and are even accumulated in enormous quantities in cancerous tissue. The diagnosis and excretion of the heavy metals, as well as organic toxins such as insecticides, preservatives and solvents, is an important part of the Paracelsus Tumour Healthcare Programme!

Not only dental heavy metals, but also dental foci and hidden dental/jaw bone infections are evaluated and treated.

Mistletoe therapy and other methods of treatment using plants (phytotherapy)

Biological strategies for attacking tumours are also used in phytotherapy (herbal medicine): since the investigations and work of Rudolf Steiner, the value of mistletoe therapy has been well known and was recognised by scientists as a result of research findings in the last decade.

The doctors at the Paracelsus Clinics have developed a very special type of mistletoe therapy which adds additional substances to the tried and tested mistletoe remedies produced by the Weleda company and which inhibit cancer in the same way. This mistletoe therapy is a unique method, the effect of which is to destroy cancer cells and at the same time stimulate the immune system!

Heat treatments / hyperthermia

Fever therapy, which has been known since ancient times, was given new impetus with the introduction of modern techniques: as a result **whole body hyperthermia** complementing **local hyperthermia (Indiba)** offers the possibility of carrying out targeted and safe treatments of cancer patients under the supervision of a physician. As the investigations of Prof. von Ardenne show, cancer cells have a reduced tolerance of heat. Tumour cells die off whilst healthy tissue remains unaffected by the surrounding temperature. On the other hand: healthy tissue and healthy defence cells react in situations where fever is present (even if artificially induced) with an increase in activity and readiness to defend the body.

The third method of heat treatment is the **infrared sauna**. In this procedure heat is produced which has a subcutaneous effect at a depth of about 5 – 8 cm and here – that is, right in the lymphatic system – stimulates the metabolism and detoxification. The patient is given an application of one of the different methods of hyperthermia on a daily basis.

Cancer and attitude to life

It is an open secret that the patient's mental state can have a considerable influence on the development and progress of cancers. A new science has been given the complicated name "psychoneuroimmunology" and is continually gaining new insights into these interrelationships. Therefore, if the cancer is to be overcome, it is not sufficient for the patient to simply undergo treatment passively. On the emotional level too, impulses for healing must be both received and given by the patient him/herself. This ancient knowledge in all advanced civilisations and religions is slowly beginning to take its place again in modern medicine. The doctors at the Paracelsus Clinics have used this type of "psychotherapy" and developed a method corresponding to the meridian system of Chinese medicine and the conclusions of Dr. Hamer which shows the patient his/her "cancer life theme". Paracelsus Clinic developed an unique psychological and energetic approach to the cancer theme with

• Kinesiology with Mr. Wolfgang Haas

• Mr. Michael Falkner's Eurythmy and future-oriented Simonton-Psychotherapy

• Evaluation of the Meridians archetype Cancer-theme

• Energetic work with our healer Mr. Peter Graus

Cancer therapy based on European Biological Medicine
The cancer therapy based on European Biological Medicine which is offered at the Paracelsus Clinics is therefore based on the following indispensable points:

1. **Nutritional therapy** with only essential substances being given. A change to food rich in bases and consistent avoidance of contaminated "modern" foodstuffs which support disease.

2. A **diet** which is completely free of allergenic foods. These are tested on an individual basis and the patient is given advice on nutrition which is appropriate to him/her. People with cancer almost always have food allergies, very frequently to the protein in cow's milk and/or hens' eggs, less frequently to wheat products. As a precaution, therefore, these are omitted completely during the Healthcare Programme. Food allergies put a tremendous strain on the immune system and as a result indirectly support the development of cancer.

3. Intensive and individually adapted **orthomolecular therapy** incorporating modern scientific findings regarding vitamins, minerals and trace elements. This also includes, for example, deacidification ther apy in the form of **alkaline infusions (= Dr. Rau's Base-Infusions)** in which relatively high doses of cell-activating trace elements and vitamins are given.

4. **Isopathic milieu therapy** according to Prof. Enderlein: this means the treatment of factors which support tumours and which are present in the blood plasma and blood cells in detectable amounts. Here dark-

field microscopy in particular is used to make a diagnosis. The Paracelsus Clinics are the only clinics to integrate Prof. Enderlein's treatment to their cancer program.

5. **Treatment of the patient's own blood** in order to strengthen the immune system, in the form of ultraviolet radiation of the blood and ozone oxygen therapy. Both treatments support the circulation and activity of the healthy blood and intracellular tissue and their ability to regenerate. At the same time, the detoxification of toxic substances (e.g. following chemotherapy and similar treatments) can be considerably improved.

6. These detoxification measures are supported by therapies of a type which support detoxification of the intestine; these reverse the displacement of the acid/base balance which always occurs in cancer patients and thus speed up the restoration of the important intestinal immune system (colonic irrigation, as well as reflorisation as introduced in Europe by the Paracelsus Clinic Lustmühle).

7. **Whole body and local hyperthermia** – as already described above – can effect an increase in the body's own defence mechanisms. The number of lymph cells and so-called macrophages increase greatly, whilst malignant and sick cells die off.

8. **Detoxification** therapies with heavy metal excretion therapies and infrared sauna and also <u>dental treatment</u>.

9. **Mistletoe therapy and enzyme therapies.**

10. **Homeopathy**. Cancer is co-caused by an energetical and constitutional weakness, which can be influed by individual high potency Homeopathy. The Paracelsus Clinic doctors took over and further developed a special technique of complex (Nosodes) and single remedy homeopathy.

These courses of treatment are supported with, for example, homeopathic remedies promoting excretion, oxygen inhalations and other procedures.

The patient is given the opportunity to rediscover his/her mental balance as a result of psychological treatment offered at the same time and to contemplate new goals of a mental and spiritual nature alongside his/her new orientation on the physical level. This complex and profound treatment can be described as unique in its compactness. By consistently carrying out all these measures and removing foci of disturbance (e.g. in collaboration with our colleagues in the dental department), it is possible within a short time not only to stop the progress of a tumour disease but also to set healing processes in motion. Patients who have already undergone conventional treatment for tumours will recover more quickly and need less medication under a properly thought out course of holistic biological treatment.

The sequence of events in the basic Paracelsus Healthcare Programme
The Paracelsus Tumour Healthcare Programme and the biological procedures used within this make it necessary to carry out a detailed examination so that we can keep our patients as safe as possible and carry out a systematic course of bio-LOGICAL treatment.

We, the physicians of the Paracelsus team, try to carry out real research into the causes of the illness and not simply to treat the symptom of cancer which appears very late on (!). We do not know all the possible causes which may lead to cancer. But we compare it to a jigsaw puzzle: the more parts we know, the clearer the picture appears, giving us the opportunity to treat in a targeted manner.

The Paracelsus Tumour Healthcare Programme therefore includes several stages

• **Diagnosis**
This is concerned with a search for foci of interference, the acid/base balance and the vitality of the blood (darkfield diagnosis). Findings from earlier investigations are of value in this context, however we always ask each patient to bring with them a recent picture (orthopantomagraph) of their teeth.

Normally a search is made at the beginning of the Healthcare Programme for foci of interference and meridian connections, using thermoregulation diagnosis; further, the vitality of the cells and the levels of antioxidants required are defined.

A special test of the vegetative tonus shows us the strength of the person's "recovery system", the parasympathetic nervous system.

- **Change of diet**
As described above, the diet of cancer patients must be rich in essential nutrients, but above all low in animal protein and free of cows' milk products. We offer a special diet which is fully adequate and rich in roughage, together with proven supporting factors (green tea, vegetable juices). We specifically support the detoxification of the liver and kidneys and – very important – prescribe polyunsaturated fatty acids.

- **Supporting treatment of foci of interference and pain**
  – Neural therapy with homeopathic and isopathic healing remedies.
  – Insufflation of the tissues with CO_2.

- **Physical and detoxification treatments**
  – Colonic irrigation
  – Local and whole body hyperthermia
  – Infrared saunas
  – Infusions of bases and vital substances / infusions for the excretion of heavy metals
  – Mistletoe therapy (the special Paracelsus Clinic Lustmühle form)
  – Massages, cupping treatments, lymph drainage (on an individual basis, according to the type of tumour)

Intensive treatment with **biological healing remedies (isopathy, immune- biology, enzyme therapy, catalyst therapy)** is begun and can be continued at home after the Healthcare Programme. In special cases we carry out **low-dose chemotherapy** which we have developed (according to Dr. Rau's method) or targeted **injection therapy** around the site of the tumour with substances which restrict the growth of tumours (prostate cancer / breast cancer).

Cost of the medical part of the Healthcare Programme
We regard every chronic illness as an individual problem – in contrast to the somewhat different views held by "conventional" medicine. Therefore before you enter our clinic we will put together a provisional

but comprehensive programme which can or must be altered as necessary during your stay according to your individual needs.

The Healthcare Programme should last for at least 2, preferably 3-4 weeks. It has been shown – as seen from the descriptions above – that it has a regenerative effect on the ground and immune system, which in cancer patients is badly disturbed. Together with the correct physical and psychological measures, it can be a real turning point – away from illness and back to health.

Dr. Thomas Rau, M.D.
Paracelsus Klinik Lustmühle,
9062 Lustmühle (bei St.Gallen)
Switzerland

Dr. Olaf Kuhnke, MD
Chief Physician
Clinica Paracelsus Al Ronc
Switzerland

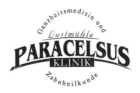

10

Causes of the development of cancer

TABLE AND SHORT EXPLANATORY TEXT
ON THE DEVELOPMENT OF CANCER:

Biological Medicine regards **cancer** as a dynamic process and never as a state. That is, cancer develops slowly and moves through different phases of degeneration down to the deterioration of the cells.

In many cases, in particular in the early stages of the cancer illness, this development can be stopped or even cancelled, if the causes of the development of cancer are eliminated.

The causes and influences, which cause the degenerative development, are only partially investigated. Many partial causes are however well-known and can be also affected. This is where **holistic, biological cancer therapy** starts.

From a holistic, biological point of view, it is of the greatest importance that each cancer patient receives a biological cancer therapy, even if he receives a parallel allopathic or alternative-medical cancer-destructive therapy. Only by removal of the cancer-favoring factors, as outlined bellow, however, can the chances of a relapse or of metastasis be decreased or avoided.

From a holistic medicine, biological point of view, metastasis or cancer relapses are new tumors, which develop because the tumor-generating factors were not eliminated.

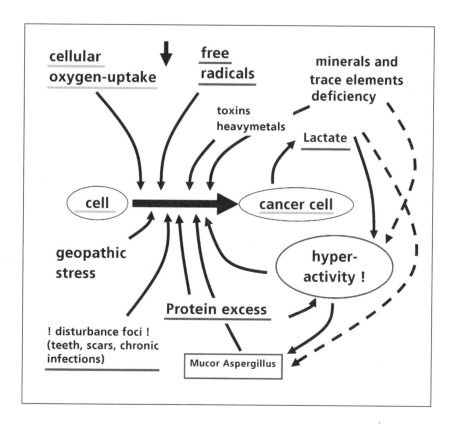

Dr. Thomas Rau, M.D.
Paracelsus Klinik Lustmühle,
9062 Lustmühle (bei St.Gallen)
Switzerland

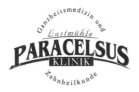

11

The Intestine, Nutrition and Health: An Explanation of Intestinal Cleansing

1. INTRODUCTION: THE IMPORTANCE OF THE INTESTINE

The intestine is by far the largest organ in the human body. The small and large intestine together measure about 6m in length and have a surface area of about 3000 m², if all the invaginations, cryptae and villi are included. On the inside, i.e. towards the intestinal lumen, the inner wall is covered with a fine **mucous membrane** which is constructed in an extremely ingenious manner. On the one hand the villous mucous membrane is able to take in nutrition, acting as a filter, but on the other hand it is also able to produce mucus and thus detoxify the body. Each day the small intestine excretes about 20 litres of mucus which ensures detoxification of the body. Apart from a few hundred millilitres, this liquid is re-absorbed back into the large intestine. However, this reabsorption requires that toxic substances are not *also* reabsorbed. Therefore there has to be an absorption system in the large intestine which holds back the material to be excreted in the intestinal lumen and prevents retoxification. This absorption system consists of the **intestinal bacteria (also called intestinal flora)** which bond with toxins and heavy metals and excrete these within the stools.

These tiny intestinal bacteria are so very numerous that the human body contains about the same number of intestinal bacteria as it has cells. As the human race has developed, they have adapted to the human body and are absolutely vitally important. The intestinal bacteria have an enormous natural ability to multiply and with their primitive life force affect the whole person. In addition the intestinal mucous membrane forms hormone – and enzyme-like substances which influence a person's ability to digest and also control the **vegetative nervous system** (serotonin, histamine, amylase, etc). The vagus or parasympathetic – that is, unconscious – nervous system also lies along the intestine and controls all our rhythmic and unconscious life functions such as breathing, heart beat, ability to recover, sleep, intestinal peristalsis, etc.

A person's true recovery is therefore very much linked with intact intestinal flora and intestinal activity! Intestinal cleansing is in many cases the most important part of a cure designed to build up the patient and aid recovery as well as to build up the immune system!

Again it is very closely linked with the intestinal flora. However, the intestine also supports the largest part of the immune system: within the mucous membrane lie the so-called "Peyer's patches" – that is, the smallest lymph cell follicles, which are present in such large numbers that the intestine therefore contains 80% of the lymphocytic immune system!

2. THE CAUSES OF A SICK INTESTINE

Incorrect diet

Nowadays food is no longer whole food. Whole food would mean that it contains all the necessary minerals, vitamins and nutritional requirements. Mostly these are greatly lacking, particularly in the case of trace elements and the essential, highly unsaturated fats. On the other hand there is mostly a massive overload of protein from animal products. This protein overload (proteins consist of amino acids) causes strong over-acidification of the organism.

Some of today's foodstuffs are of inferior quality and produced too quickly, and plants simply do not have the time to absorb from the soil the important trace elements. This results in a lack of essential trace elements such as manganese, molybdenum, selenium, chromium, etc., which are particularly important for the intactness of the intestine. This deficiency is reinforced even more strongly in the case of food from animal sources, as nowadays even cattle lack trace elements, particularly manganese and molybdenum, to a great degree.

This is why, at the beginning of your treatment with us to build up your body, you will be given these substances as additional remedies in order to replenish what is lacking. Then later a correct diet will perhaps be sufficient to maintain the level of trace elements in your body.

Another frequent problem in nutrition is the lack of polyunsaturated fatty acids, which are of the greatest importance for all nerve functions and the brain as well as for the building up of all the cell membranes.

People today generally take the view that fats are bad, so they try to eat as little fatty food as possible. By doing this they reduce their intake of the bad, saturated fats which only overload the body. But generally this is done in the wrong way, by eating only low-fat meat, fish and a low-fat diet, instead of adding the important fats. This mistake comes mainly from the fact that people no longer use oil.

Cold-pressed vegetable oils are the specific sources of the unsaturated fatty acids which are important for life. We should have an intake of approximately 30 grams per day of these high-quality oils! And so in our diet you will be given raw salads with oils. Olive oil, wheatgerm oil, linseed oil and evening primrose oil are particularly good. We even recommend that you take a dessertspoonful of these oils each day. Grapeseed oil, with a very neutral taste and very good for you, is also well-tried and tested and of high quality, as too is sesame oil which however has a very particular taste. By adding unsaturated fatty acids to your diet you will support your body's own synthesis of hormones. This is particularly important for people in the middle and older age-groups.

Preservatives

Many foodstuffs are made to last longer by the addition of preservatives and stabilisers: for example, all ready-made drinks, sweet drinks, long-life bread, tinned and vacuum-packed foods. These preservatives are supposed to prevent bacteria or fungi developing on the foods. But the problem is then that these preservatives can also do the same thing in the human body, particularly in the vital intestinal flora – that is, alter the intestinal flora! It is of the greatest importance to eat only foodstuffs which are fresh and free of preservatives, preferably so-called "wholefoods".

Too little liquid or the wrong type

Everything that you take into your body which then leaves it as part of the detoxification process must pass through the barrier of the intestinal mucous membrane in a dissolved form. It is therefore of the greatest importance that you drink water, which enables all the work of transportation and dissolving in your body. For this purpose the body needs about 2 to 3 litres of pure water daily!

All "drinks" which contain proteins, fats and carbohydrates are useless and should count as foodstuffs, as they cannot carry out the functions of dissolving and transportation. We need water to clean the body and to keep all the life functions flowing and dynamic. Would you do *your* washing using milk or fruit juice? Milk and fruit juices are not drinks and we advise against them totally! Fruit juices can be taken in very small amounts *before* meals to stimulate the production of digestive juices. A maximum of ½ a wine glass full before breakfast or lunch. No more!

Drink pure water. Drink between mealtimes so as not to dilute the digestive juices. Drink the water at a temperature which feels warm to the hand or even hot. Teas are permitted and they can even strengthen the metabolic function, e.g. lime blossom, peppermint or lavender tea. But most of the water that you drink should be in the form of pure water!

In both the Paracelsus Clinica Al Ronc and the Paracelsus Klinik Lustmühle we provide water which has been prepared with special purifiers and "energising" apparatus and which is significantly better for the body in various different ways: purified from suspended matter, excess protein build-up and toxins and also to a great extent free of heavy metals. In the machines which we have set up (Singer water ionizers in Al Ronc and oxygenating and magnetizing water machines in Lustmühle) the energy content and molecular structure clusters of the water are also improved, which is why these types of water are said to be better at removing toxic products and acting as a means of transport.

Medications

Medications can be extremely bad for the intestinal mucous membrane and in particular the intestinal bacteria: antibiotics destroy the intestinal bacteria and in the long term lead to the development of false bacteria in forms which are known as amoebic – that is, lacking cell walls. Thus over a long period of time antibiotics also lead to internal poisoning, as the normal intestinal bacteria can no longer act as toxin absorbers. In addition to having a proper diet, people who are prescribed antibiotics therefore need specific remedies which build up the intestinal bacteria again: the doctors in Al Ronc and the Paracelsus Klinik Lüstmuhle use the isopathic remedies from the German company Sanum-Kehlbeck.

Food allergy: the cause of many immunological problems

Food allergies are the most frequent hidden causes of chronic illnesses. They have their roots in early childhood, when the mother stops breastfeeding the infant. For various reasons infants are often given cow's milk instead of mother's milk. At this age the child's pancreas is not yet fully developed and cannot cope with strange protein. The cow's milk proteins are therefore not broken down sufficiently, and the molecules which pass across the intestinal mucous membrane – which is still too porous at this age – are too big. These large protein molecules then act as allergens and overload the young child's lymphatic system (to be precise, the above-mentioned Peyer's patches).

The triggering allergen in cow's milk is beta-lactoglobulin, which to date neither the chemical industry nor the milk industry has ever been able to separate out of milk. All cow's milk products such as butter, yoghurt, cheese, etc. and even margarine with 2 % cow's milk contain this allergen. The infant does not show an allergic reaction immediately; only when he is older does he get rheumatism or skin problems or respiratory tract problems, etc. In the first nine months of life infants should also not be given any fresh fruit or vegetables, because this can also lead to a strain on the pancreas.

Adults who acquired this allergy as babies mostly show absolutely no symptoms if they eat and drink milk products but instead develop problems of the immune system or chronic diseases. However, even as adults they can be greatly helped by a diet which is free of cow's milk.

The function of the pancreas can also be improved in adulthood by a diet without cow's milk but rich in minerals and if the patient gradually goes over to a diet with fresh vegetables and vegetable proteins. These limitations are maintained until any secondary symptoms of the food allergy, such as skin, joint and respiratory tract problems, have cleared up. Afterwards these foodstuffs can again be included in the menu plan with a reduction in their quantity.

Just by the way; before and after pregnancy the mother-to-be should gradually reduce her consumption of cow's milk products.

Chronic constipation

Chronic constipation is one of the most frequent complaints of older patients and (like chronic sleeping difficulties) is almost always a symptom of a reduction in the intestinal flora, a reduction in the surface area of the intestinal mucous membrane and exhaustion of the parasympathetic (vagus) nervous system. Chronic constipation can mostly be improved within a short time if the intestinal flora are built up with the right sort of food (see the Paracelsus nutritional guidelines below) and the parasympathetic nervous system is stimulated. That again happens with trace elements and neural therapy, but also by having the right sort of drinks.

Chronic constipation is often the joint cause of chronic intoxications, as in cases of constipation in the large intestine too many toxins are digested by the body and then overload the liver. This strain on the liver again leads to fatigue, depression and sleeping problems.

A special case: leaky gut syndrome

More and more frequently we see the problem of leaky gut syndrome which the patient never notices in the intestine but always only because of chronic toxic problems: tiredness, tendency to allergies, problems with sleeping and concentration, etc. The problem lies in the fact that in these patients oversized molecules and allergens have been taken into the body and thereby bring the body to a continuous state of overload of the immune system. The diagnosis can be made by means of differentiated stool tests (ortho-analytic stool health check) or hair mineral analysis or darkfield microscopy. There is even a test in orthodox medicine that points to this: the lactose/mannitol test, which to be sure does not give conclusive results on the porosity of relatively small-moleculed allergens. But very little is still known about the disorder, although it is assumed that it can have a big influence on the immune system.

For the holistic Paracelsian doctor, however, this diagnosis is of great importance, as this disease can be improved or healed further by diet and with Sanum remedies and trace elements.

3. THE CONSEQUENCES OF A SICK INTESTINE

Civilisation diseases connected with intestinal problems

Excess acid in the organism
A diet which is too rich in protein and contains sugar leads to an increase in the production of acid throughout the body and to many secondary diseases:

Mycoses: Excess of acid in the body, especially in the connective tissues, favours the growth of fungi. The consumption of alcohol, analgesics, antibiotics, hormones, psychopharmacologic drugs etc. can support this fungal growth even more. The acid-base balance can be regulated and the fungus brought to a lower stage of development by means of a suitable diet and additional isopathic remedies in the initial stages, without destroying the intestinal flora at the same time.

Constipation: A feeling of fullness, diarrhoea, constipation or enterogastritis can be a sign of allergy to cow's milk or hens' eggs, but also a sign of a reduction in the intestinal flora. The regulation of the digestive system is extremely important and the intestinal mucous membrane, pancreas and liver must work well together; i.e. initially at least the pancreas and liver must be supported with remedies.

The joints: Allergies to cow's milk or hens' eggs can also manifest themselves as rheumatic pains in the ankle joints, knees, hips, shoulders, elbows and wrists. Orthodox medical laboratory tests will not necessarily find anything specific.

Circulation: A rise in the pulse rate, sudden fainting, a red face, increased sweating, etc. point to strain on the circulation. Burning eyes, itching of the neck, sneezing attacks, an increase in the breathing rate (possibly combined with fear) are also some of the forms in which one recognises food allergies. The secondary consequences include hypertonia, coronary heart disease, angina pectoris and other heart problems.

Obesity: Because of a reaction which is dependent on histamine, hidden food allergens block the burning up of fat and thus can prevent fat being burnt up even in periods of fasting. A strict low-allergen diet is therefore extremely important, even in people who are able to reduce the fatty tissue. The Paracelsus Kliniks offer initially both low-allergen fasting diets and differentiated and individual testing for food allergies with immunoglobulin tests, thermoregulation diagnosis and bioresonance testing.

Problems of the immune system
As described above, the intestine is the largest organ of the immune system and contains 80% of an adult's lymph follicles. It is this lymphocytic immunity which is largely reliant on the intestine being healthy. An upset in the system of white blood cells (leucocytes and lymphocytes) is accompanied by a reduction in the number of "killer cells" and phagocytes and thus also reduces the body's defences against viral diseases and cancer.

As a special feature of our therapy we also have particular biological remedies for this weakness of the lymph cells: thymo preparations, xenogen peptide and Rebas, a specific remedy to build up the Peyer's patches of the intestine.

Toxic overloads
These can occur if the intestine becomes more porous (see above) or if there is constipation. But the most frequent cause of chronic toxic overload is the reduction in the normal number of intestinal flora. The intestinal bacteria bond with poisons which are excreted from the body into the intestine and carry them in the stools out of the body. A diet which builds up the intestinal flora automatically also supports the detoxification of the body. This diet must be low in allergens and rich in

minerals and plant fibres – in other words it must contain finely grated raw foods and high-quality oils.

Chronic tiredness

The so-called "chronic fatigue syndrome" is always an illness with many facets of which the individual causes are combined in a very individual way. However, there are always problems with the intestinal flora and the lymphocytic immune system. The reduction in the intestinal flora leads to a lowering of the body's ability to recover and weakening of the parasympathetic nervous system. Infections with viruses which cause chronic fatigue, such as the Epstein Barr virus, are only a consequence of something else. Chronic fatigue syndrome is a disease of the immune system and intestine, and is often significantly improved within a few weeks or months by a broad-based course of immune therapy and the building up of the intestine, combined with our infusions.

4. WAYS TO CLEANSE THE INTESTINE

A change of diet

Eating should be a pleasure and we ought to take the time we need for it. A healthy diet begins with chewing one's meals for a long time. This allows sufficient saliva to form in order for digestion to be supported. The saliva itself contains digestive enzymes (amylase / disaccharase), and chewing stimulates the pancreas by means of a reflex reaction. Every mouthful must be chewed 15 – 20 times. Everything that you swallow should enter the stomach in the form of fine broth.

Drinking with meals lessens this enzyme stimulation and should be avoided. Drink between meals – but very little with meals! Every excessive addition to your food is indigestible. When you are stressed and tired, your organs also do not function at their best and the digestive system is put under strain. The main meal of the day should be breakfast, the evening meal should be small and easily digested. No fruit in the evening as it can lead to fermentation.

Cleansing of the intestine is indicated when the patient has not been having an ideal diet over a long period, for whatever reason. Children are also a target group, and in such cases it is best if a change of diet is introduced for the whole family out of solidarity with the child and for everyone's benefit. At the beginning the change is awkward, but even after a few days the patient will notice an improvement.

Diet in Greek means a "way of life"

A "diet" in the sense of a change of nutrition is necessary if

- As a child you were not breastfed for the first 9 months and were fed cow's milk and cow's milk products or hen's eggs and hen's egg products from an early age. Allergic diseases of the skin, respiratory tract and sinuses can be the result of this

- You suffer from recurrent diarrhoea, constipation or wind

- You suffer from chronic illnesses

- You have remote problems, i.e. if disturbed intestinal flora indirectly upset different organs and as a result cause eczema, fungal infections, psoriasis, neurodermatitis or strong acne on the skin; bronchial asthma, bronchitis, inflammation of the sinuses in the respiratory tract; or arthritis, gout or rheumatism in the joints

- Detoxification and drainage are indicated, for example in the case of coproliths (faecal stones), old food residues, overload of heavy metals with amalgam, palladium, mercury, aluminium and other poisons

After 14 days of a change of diet you will notice a change in your body. If the result is not sweeping, complementary medical remedies should also be given, such as vitamins and minerals, as well as isopathic remedies to stimulate the immune system. At the beginning of the changeover, personal allergens and primary allergens (cow's milk and hen's egg preparations) should be completely omitted from the diet. The menu provided in the Paracelsus Kliniks, in particular in the Clinica Al Ronc, is designed according to the very latest knowledge as described above and can help all patients with allergies, disorders of the immune system, and digestive, circulatory and heart problems. Our food supports the building up of the body and is therefore a "must" for people who need to recover.

Colonic irrigation

In the Lustmühle and Al Ronc Paracelsus Kliniks there has been further development of a specialised system of colonic irrigation which:

- Uses lavages to clean the large intestine up as far as the small intestine, with all its thousands of evaginations. In these crypts there are often toxic crusts which are years old and even parasites and foci of inflammation. If the irrigation is carried out carefully, it can even be ideal for patients with colitis or recurrent diverticulitis! In such cases, however, the colonic irrigation must always be accompanied by our flora repopulation and intensive biological therapy and diet

- Stimulates the parasympathetic nervous system by means of very soft, deep abdominal massages

- Builds up the intestinal flora again by follow-up irrigation with special bacterial solutions, the composition of which matches that of the human symbiotic flora. These bacterial solutions are a specialised development which is exclusive to the Paracelsus Kliniks

- Detoxifies the body through the osmotic effect of the irrigation

- It is advisable to have this colonic irrigation once or twice a week during the cure

Building up of the flora with medication

A particular speciality of the Paracelsus Kliniks. The building up of the good, symbiotic intestinal flora is supported by means of a mixture of isopathic remedies and neural therapy applied to quite specific points of the intestine.

Immune stimulation

The most important point in the building up of the intestine and of immune stimulation is the omission from the diet of food allergens, mostly products containing cow's milk and hen's eggs.

This restores the Peyer's patches and as a secondary benefit also strengthens the intestinal mucous membrane. Further immune stimulation of the intestinal system can be achieved by the trace elements selenium, molybdenum, vitamins A, B6 and B12, Biotin and vitamin E. In addition the patients are generally also prescribed special bacterial remedies produced by the Sanum company: Utilin and Recarcin capsules, generally at a dosage of 1 of each per week.

A healthy immune system can be guaranteed
only by having a healthy intestine!

A diet to cleanse the intestine, build up the immune system and reduce acid:
the Paracelsus Al Ronc diet
The diet at the Al Ronc Paracelsus health centre is based on years of experience and is suitable for almost everybody. It follows strictly the dietary rules laid down by Dr. Thomas Rau, M.D., and the hypoallergenic diet designed by Dr. Konrad Werthmann, M.D.

This diet

- Strengthens and relieves the strain on the immune system, as the common allergens are for the most part omitted

- Supports the building up of the intestinal mucous membrane within 6 – 12 weeks and of the intestinal flora within about 3 weeks

- Brings about a significant improvement to the patient's well-being and to their day/night rhythm within 3 weeks

- Leads in the long term to optimisation of weight (amazingly, people who are overweight lose weight, and those who are underweight gain weight as the metabolism is normalised)

- Leads within a few weeks to the removal of excess acid from the body

- Strengthens the Peyer's lymph follicles and strengthens the immune system

Principles of the diet used in the Paracelsus Clinica Al Ronc

- No meat, except occasionally some fish: meat from warm-blooded animals, in particular that of mammals, contains protein (in Prof. Enderlein's words, "endobiontic proteins") which in the human body can develop into bacteria but in particular can also cause the blood to thicken.

- No meat as it is very acidic.

- No white sugar or products containing white sugar. All sweet food is prepared using sweeteners such as honey, concentrated extract of pear, agave syrup, Stevia, etc.

- Strictly no products containing cow's milk, on allergenic grounds. The calcium which is supposed to be so important in such milk is more than compensated for by the correct choice of calcium-rich vegetables!

- The drinks which are freely available between mealtimes are teas, with different types selected each day.

- The emphasis is on the morning and lunchtime meals. In the evenings only small, light meals are served.

- In the morning we recommend the Paracelsus basic soup, a vegetable broth which is very rich in minerals and very alkaline. (The recipe is given in the paper on Chronic Hypoglycemia).

- The addition of sufficient unsaturated fatty acids is considered extremely important, so unless required you will not be given any oil rations.

- About one-third of the vegetables should be eaten raw, preferably finely grated. The cellulose fibres of the raw vegetables provide nourishment for the intestinal flora and clean the intestine mechanically.

What you should avoid

Cow's milk and products containing cow's milk: Milk, cheese, whey, margarine which contains butter, yoghurt, quark, bifidus, kefir, ice cream, milk chocolate. Even in Biological Medicine circles there are different opinions regarding cream and butter, which are both prepared from the fat of cow's milk (without protein). In the Paracelsus Clinic Al Ronc they are not used, instead the valuable vitamins and fats which they contain are replaced by oils and vegetables. (Sheep's and goat's milk cheeses are permitted: Roquefort, peccorino, etc)

Hen's eggs and products containing hen's eggs: Breaded products, mayonnaise, French dressing, dough products made with egg, ready-prepared soups in cartons, tarts, blancmange, mousse, icing, cakes, sweet biscuits, Ovaltine. Because of frequent allergies to hens' eggs which would help to build up the patient's strength (e.g. poached, or boiled for 3 minutes), quail's eggs are used instead.

Pork and all pork products: Roast pork, sausages and salami, ham, bacon, ravioli, cold meats

Rabbit, venison and other game: Meat from hunted animals contains histamine and can cause allergies

Shellfish and other fish, tinned fish: Tuna, mackerel, lobster, crayfish, shrimps and prawns, mussels, snails. The "fruits of the sea" often contain heavy metals, and certain varieties also contain a lot of histamine.
Nuts: Peanuts, peanut oil, walnuts, coconuts, muesli bars, multi-grain full corn bread.

Citrus fruits: Lemons, limes, oranges, mandarins/satsumas, grapefruit. Occasionally eating a grapefruit for breakfast or in Bircher muesli is allowed.

Soft drinks: CocaCola (including diet Coke), lemonade, Orangina, Pepita, ready-made iced tea, Rivella

Coffee: Not more than 1 – 2 cups per day, making sure that it is organic coffee. Coffee attacks the regulatory mechanism of the renin and angiotensin and this has an effect on the excretion of water, dehydrates and is acidic. During intensive phases of therapy (fasting, detoxifying, etc) coffee should therefore not be drunk at all.

Various: Ketchup, mustard, kiwi, sugar, nicotine, large quantities of rose hip and camomile tea.

An important reminder is that from 5.00 pm onwards you should not eat raw fruit and vegetables, and never have your drinks cold!

Recommended protein foods in a vegetarian diet
The question is frequently asked: how then can the missing proteins be supplied in a meat- and milk-free diet? The answer – valuable plant proteins, which are also mostly alkaline:

- Linseed, beans, peas

- Potatoes

- Sweetcorn

- Chestnuts

- Avocados

- The seeds of various types of plants

- Quorn or textured vegetable protein (TVP / mianjin / seitan)

- Millet or cereal grains (pil-pil)

It should be taken into account that the "normal" average European person eats far too much protein and that this is the cause of many diseases. The ideal intake of protein is about 40 grams per day (as opposed to about 120 g/day average consumption!). With a varied vegetarian diet one can therefore easily get enough high-quality protein which at the same time is a much better "carrier" of trace elements and vitamins, as well as saving energy.

Helpful tips and alternatives to forbidden foods

Milk products: Soya milk, soya cream, soya pudding, soya yoghurt, soya drinks, goat's milk, sheep's milk, rice milk

Butter: Margarine which does not contain cow's milk: e.g. Vitabiosa, Eden and Vitaquell

Cheese: Sheep's cheese, goat's cheese, peccorino, Roquefort, feta, and soya cheese

Eggs: Quail's eggs, duck eggs, turkey eggs
For batter coatings: mix sheep's or soya milk with some flour or mix together 1 tbsp. rice flour with 1 tbsp. water or coat with pure beef dripping (not pork dripping)

Fish: Eat fish at best 1 – 2 times a week. No shellfish or crustaceans (prawns) or tinned fish.

Seeds: Sunflower, pumpkin, sesame seeds and cashew nuts (= seeds)

Vegetables, fruits: Use seasonal products: these are valuable, tasty and cheap.
Of course we recommend naturally pickled vegetables such as sauerkraut in small quantities but taken regularly

Oils: Cold pressed / virgin oils such as olive oil, sunflower oil, grapeseed oil, etc. Wheatgerm oil

Mayonnaise: DIP sauce powder as a vegetarian replacement without egg yolk and protein. Keeps well.

Sauces: Read the ingredients named on the packaging. The use of fresh products is preferable.

Soups: Meat-free vegetable bouillon as a base for soup, cooking dough products and rice, available in health food shops. (Nahrin)

Cereals: Various types of rice, sweetcorn, barley, couscous, quinoa, oats, semolina. Important: millet, sweetcorn (maize) and rice contain no gluten and are therefore permitted foods for all people with an allergy to cereals: millet bread and maize bread are available in specialist shops.

Dough products: Italian pasta made of 100% durum wheat semolina and water, e.g. Barilla, Tipo Napoli

Sweeteners: Honey, concentrated pear syrup, maple syrup, stevia leaves for drinks, and sweets: sorbet made only of fruit juice and sugar, soya creams of all types (except nut)

Vegetarian specialities: Tartex, Seitan (TVP), etc

Baby products: Milupa SOM (soya milk) and porridge, Humana SL and porridge, or Galactina Mamina Junior Bio (soya- based only).

Dr. Thomas Rau, M.D.
Paracelsus Klinik Lustmühle,
9062 Lustmühle (bei St.Gallen)
Switzerland

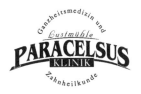

12

The Reflorastation of the Small and Large Intestines

ON THE IMPORTANCE AND TECHNIQUE OF THE REFLORISTATION OF INTESTINAL FLORA, AND IMMUNE STIMULATION

Table of contents:

Appendix:

THE REFLORASTATION OF THE SMALL AND LARGE INTESTINES AT THE PARACELSUS KLINIK, ACCORDING TO DR. MED. THOMAS RAU

Introduction

Humans have more intestinal bacteria than own cells. The intestine bacteria are an important "internal organ", since they have completely adapted themselfs to humans and fulfill very important functions. They are mainly responsible for the detoxification of the body as a whole, and the immune system in particular. Furthermore, they make possible the admission of substances to the body, such as pro-vitamines or trace-elements – which are otherwise only partly absorbed by the body with difficulty – since they de-metabolise them or bind them organically,.

The following can lead to a reduction of intestinal flora in the small and large intestines:

- All antibiotics
- Anti-acidity agents of the newer generation (gastric acid blockers)
- Laxatives
- Nikotin abuse
- Preservatives in the nutrition
- Wrong nutrition, i.e. lack of vegetables and raw food and too much meat
- Food allergies lead to intestinal atrophy and thus to a reduction of the intestinal flora.

The reflorastation of the intestines is one of the most important measures with all immune disturbances and with all toxically caused suffering. In particular however, all tendancies to infection must be treated by means of regeneration.

The reflorastation of the intestines is developed on two stages:
1. The reflorastation of the small intestines
2. The reflorastation of the large intestines

THE REFLORASTATION OF THE SMALL INTESTINES

Nowadays, reductions in anaerobic acidic flora – like Bacteroides, Lactophilus and Bifidus hominis – are nearly always present,. More rarely, actualy harmfull bacteria like Pseudomonas and Klebsiellen are present. This, again, is usually caused by a weakness of the intestinal mucosa and the anaerobic flora. Candida, however, grows practically only in humans with high heavy metal levels. With parasites or dysbacteria, we refer the reader to the separate additional therapy plan in the appendix.

It is wrong to treat such bacteria with anti-means such as antibiotics or antimykotics but rather one must strengthen, on the one hand, the environment of the intestinal mucosa and, on the other hand, strengthen the correct intestinal flora.

Preparations for the substitution of the intestinal flora in the small intestines (can be used initially for some weeks) :

- **Lactobact** powder: 2x1 teaspoons, before or between meals, for 4-6 weeks
- **Probiotic** caps.: 3x1, after 2 weeks reduce to 2x1 , between meals
- **Bioflorin** caps.: 3x1, in each case before meals, after 1 week reduce to 1/day
- **Symbioflor** dr.: 3x15 drops, on a long-term basis, to be taken with a little water

One can also – esp. with immune disturbances and with children with a tendancy to infections – begin at first with **Pro-Symbioflor** or **Colibiogen-Kinder**, whereby then a careful, slowly increasing dosage should be selected: beginning with 3x3, then daily increasing around a drop, to 3 x 10 dr.. Then on to **Symbioflor 1**. We rarely use **Symbioflor**

2, Mutaflor or other preparations for the flora of the large intestine. In our opinion, the intestinal flora of the small intestines should be regenerated rectaly.

Plan for regenerating the intestine environment, and thus the actual long-term refloristation of intestinal flora:

Gradual increase with isopathic **Sanum** cures:

- three weeks long **Fortakehl**
- begin after one week, also for 3 weeks: **Pefrakehl**
- beginning after a further week, then for several months: **Sankombi** drop, 2-3 x 10 dr.

This bacterial therapy is supported with the bacterial immune stimulation products of **Sanum**:

- alternating 1 caps. per week, **Recarcin** (Bac. Firmus) D6 caps and
- **Utilin** (Bac.subtilis) D6 caps. (s. appendix: on simple immune stimulation)

This therapy with **Sanum** cures should be followed for several months.

Additionally, we advise to do the flushings of the large intestine, as recommended on the next page and the regeneration of intestinal flora, once per 1-3 weeks, altogether approx.. 4-12 X (s. article The reflorastation of the large intestines).

THE REFLORASTATION OF THE LARGE INTESTINES
ACCORDING TO DR. MED. TH. RAU
AND DR. V. BOWMANN

Introduction

The intestinal flora of the large intestine has a different function than that of the small intestine. It has, apart from the immune component functions, esp. the function of toxin absorption and elimination of harmful substances, which should not be re-absorbed from the large intestine back into the body. The ileocecal valve separates the two milia of the ileum from the colon. Bacteria of the small intestine are found only in small numbers in the large intestine. The opposite is also true. Therefore, it is also more effective to develop the intestinal flora of the large intestine rectaly.

The best methods to accomplish this are **Colon Hydrotherapy** and the **"Colon Reflorisierung"** (according to V. Bowman):

Long-term, the intestinal flora of the large intestines can also be developed with Sanum therapie, nutrition and algae:

- **Mucokehl** D3 sup., 2 x per week, one suppository in the evening, rectaly. (Mucokehl is normally a morning medicine, if taken orally. We are concerned, in this case however, with the treatment of the rektum and the liver, over the entero-hepatischen cycle. These organs regenerate at night) **Mucedokehl** D3 sup. 2 x per week a sup. in the evening. **Exmykehl** sup., once per week a sup. in the evening (esp. for Candida problems and with flatulence)

- **Algae**: Chlorella Paracelsus (or a Spirulina preparation, e.g. Burgerstein Spirulina) 3x4-6 tabl., taken between meals with much liquid, unfolds its absorbative effect and binds toxins and heavy metals. The dosage can be individually reduced or also increased, esp. for heavy metals. Reduce by flatulence.

- **Okubasan** drops (Sanum), 3x10-15 drops. Okoubasan is a marvelous cure, a vegetable tannin, which works with dysbiosis, flatulence, parasites and esp. with a dietary induced change of the flora (small and large intestine). It is esp. to be taken with all foreign journeys and with frequent eating out. With each acute dysbacterial intestinal illness or intestinal irritation, it can be taken for some days in much higher dosage: 6-8 x 10-15 drops (see also "Paracelsus Parasite -Therapy")

- **Molybdenum** (Burgerstein molybdenum, tabl. @ 100mcgr.) 1 tabl per day, in the evening. Molybdenum is an important trace element, which is very frequently deficient because of modern agricultural methods. It activates the xanthine and sulfatide sulfatide-oxidasen, which, on the one hand, activate urine acid production and anti-oxydant processes and, on the other hand, supports the elimination of toxic sulfates, which can then be excreted over the intestines. Esp. meat eaters need this trace element. It favours the formation of the walls of intestinal bacteria.

- **Nutrition**: Without change of diet, no change of intestinal flora! Unfortunately, there are hardly any generally accepted dietary instructions. We refer however to the information sheet "Simple dietary guidelines", which leads to the regeneration of the intestinal environment and the acid–base regulation.

Important components for the regeneration of intestinal flora in the large intestines are the consume of finely grated vegetables, esp. carrots, zucchini, & sellerie. Caution is required with all grain products, which work today, due to the very high gluten content, for many humans as allergens. Milk and all cow's milk products must be avoided as far as possible. Only exceptions with sour milk products, but only few, permited. Cow's milk is today's main allergen!!

COLON HYDROTHERAPY

The intestinal flushings are an extremely beneficial measure for the improvement of intestinal peristalsis and the regeneration of intestinal flora. The main effect of the colon hydrotherapy lies in the deep, careful abdominal massage and not in the rinsing effect by the induced water. The abdominal massage leads to a stimulation of the parasympathetic nervous system, the vagal nervous system. The parasympathetic nervous system stimulates the general regeneration of the organism, hormonal production (esp. progesterone and testosterone, as well as melatonine) as well as intestinal peristalsis and bile secretion.
Colon hydrotherapies have a very regenerative effect. They should be carried out systematically:

Frequency: every 3-14 days, altogether 6 -12-times.

Previous to the colon hydrotherapy, magnesium sulfate (epsom salt) can be taken orally, _ – 1 tblsp. in the morning, in 2-3 glasses warm water. Anyhow, the intake of much liquid is very important.

The colon hydrotherapy should take 45-60 minutes. The lukewarm water is to be induced in a continuous stream. Under fine, vibrating massages, the water is worked up to the iliocecal valve. The return flow valve does not need to be closed, too much pressure is strictly to be avoided and painful. If the colon hydrotherapy is used in such a manner, it is also the therapy of choice with diverticulitis, colitis, etc..

Following the colon hydrotherapy, we advise the regeneration of intestinal flora according to Bowann. See next article: a measure to faster regeneration of the whole large intestine with the correct combinations of human intestinal bacteria.

THE REFLORASTATION OF THE LARGE INTESTINES ACCORDING TO MRS. VICKY BOWMAN

Practical procedure

In co-operation with Mrs. Vicky Bowman, PhD., of Arizona, we introduced, as first in Europe, a method in which, directly after the colon hydrotherapy, the correct intestinal bacteria are introduced. They then spread, due to capillary action, over the whole colon and after an intensive multiplication over 7-14 days, realize a recovery of the colon flora, if the above pieces of dietary advice are kept, at least during this time.

The **Bowman-Reflorastation-Bulk** is a powder of freez-dried bacteria, manufactured by enterprises licensed for pure bacteria products in the USA. It contains the tremendous number of 15 billion bacteria per tea spoon of powder. The bacteria contain 15 different bacterial sorts, which should be present in the human large intestine, in approximately normal quantitative proportions.

Application of the reflorastation:
After final colon hydrotherapy and following repeated bowel movements or passing of water, the patient lies again on the colon couch.

Preparation.

one takes:

- 1 measuring spoon (1 accumulated tea spoon) bacteria powder (the Reflorastation Bulk comes in a box of 500gr powder, which must be kept dry and cool)
- 1 glass container with catch (preserving jar)
- 1 disposable catheter, 30-40 cm long
- 1 60ml syringe, which fits on the disposable catheter
- Lubricating gel from Johnson & Johnson (or other water-soluble sliding gels)
- Lukewarm tap water

1 measuring spoon (or 1 tea spoon) bacterial mixture with approx. 30-40 ml lukewarm tap water vigerously shaken in a preserving jar, until it dissolves completely. Thus the freez-dried bacteria are activated. This solution is drawn up into a 60ml syringe.

After the colon hydrotherapy, the intestines are emptied again at the WC and then the refloristasion begins:

The patient lies on his left side. One spreads a lubricant on the catheter and leads this carefully approx.. 20 cm into the rectum. Now one inserts the bacterial solution (30-40ml) slowly into the intestine. The catheter is then pulled out slowly and the patient closes his sigmoid strongly. The patient must remain lying 1-2 minutes on his left side, so that the rectum and sigmoid are moistened. Then the patient turns slowly into the upside-down position and builds a "bridge" or one gives him a cushion under his bottom, so that the solution can flow up the colon descendes. That takes, again, 1-2 minutes. Then the pat. turns on the right side and stays several minutes again in this way. Then he can rise and try not go, if possible, for _-1 hour to the toilet.

After the refloristation, the patient generally feels a change of the fecal quality for some days, often experiancing flatulance. Rarely, a warming or a fever feeling can also arise on the 1st. or 2nd. day. Altogether, however, most patients experience a clear energy increase. A physician or therapist should initiate the indication.

(Source of supply of the Refloristation bacteria, from the USA manufacturer directly: Victoria Bowmann, Dr.H.M., 16034 N.23rd.Place, Phoenix, AZ 85022, E-Mail: VBowmann@aol.com, or fax 001-602-788-7557)

APPENDIX 1: THE PARACELSUS PARASITE THERAPY

Since the work of Dr. Hulda Clarck of the USA, the topic of the parasitosis in holistic medicine has become much discussed and the therapy according to Clark, with wermut, walnut and carnation preparations, well known. The treatment of dysbacteria, more tumorous or generally abdominal problems with only this threefold combination is, however, dubious and must always be based on a clinical diagnosis and must always be followed up with a holistic medicine therapy.

The companies SANUM and CERIUM offer medicines, which, in our experience usually work better than the overpaid phytotherapeutica specified above. The following plan " Paracelsus parasite therapy" has proved itself, in combination with the cures otherwise described, or also alone. It is very successful with the therapy of non-specific abdominal complaints and dyspepsia.

- **Okubasan** is a tanning agent and replaces walnut
- **Absinthium** of CERIUM is a very good choleretic
- **Leptospermusan** has a very good effect in changing the redox-potential and cell-membrane potential and works against the probably membrane-changing toxic effect of the parasites, which is why it is very suitable also for tumor patients as a secondary therapy.

APPENDIX 2: THE PARACELSUS SIMPLE IMMUNE STIMULATION PLAN

Immune stimulation should take place individually and related to the reasons for the immune weakness.most frequently, heavy metal toxicity is the cause of immune weakness, as well as immune weakness from electromagnetic fields or chronic viruses.

The focused immune stimulation with thymus or misteltoe preparations must take place individually and also according to the initial lymphatic situation.

The following **simple immune stimulation** is a basic therapy, which is very recommendable for all forms of **infectious tendencies, chronic tiredness** and **immune weaknesses,** but also, **allergies,** also for children.

An immune friendly diet always belongs to immune stimulation, which omits all main allergens:

Nutrition in immune regeneration:
- **no cow's milk products and cow's milk beverages**
- **few chicken egg foods**
- **no or few nut foods**
- **hold back strongly with all wheat products (glutin)**

Medicines
- **Utilin D6 Kps (bacillus subtilis) 1 Kps per week**
- **Recarcin D6 caps. (bacillus firmus) 1 cap. per week** the two caps. are taken on different days, with a completely empty stomach, at best, early in the morning or late at night.

After 6 weeks:
- **Utilin S D6 caps. (Mycobakterium phlei) 1 cap. per week**
- **Rebas D4 caps.**: at the beginning, during 1-2 weeks 1-2 caps. per day, then 2x1 per week
- **CERIUM Echinacea (Alcea) dr., 3x4-5 dr. per day**
- **Sankombi dr., 10 dr. per day**, wet in the mouth and then swallow.

<u>Note</u>: never use Echinacea constantly! Always use as an interval therapy. This has validity for all immune stimulators, therefore use rather immune modulators.

This therapy is taken during 1-2 months, then repeated 2 x per year.

Appendix to this article: Paracelsus parasite cure/simple Diaetanleitung/Diaetanleitung: which may be eaten/Darmflora structure

APPENDIX 2: THE PARACELSUS SIMPLE IMMUNE STIMULATION PLAN

Main paradigms:

- Parasitosis is expression of a dysbiosis / a terrain disturbance
- Parasitosis is usually laboratory-chemically not provable
- Parasitosis is a chronic problem with immune disturbance
- Parasitosis leads to toxic load (metabolic by-products)
- Parasitosis leads to systemic problems

Proof:

- Stool cultures with difficulty, since nests, usually negative
- IgE frequently increased / Eosinophile Granulocyten frequently increases
- Serology usually negative, does not say anything

Alternative medical proof:

- <u>Dryed Layer Blood test</u>: toxic lakune / lack of trace elements
- Darkfield microscopy: symplasts, very large bacterial forms
- Hair mineral analysis: indication of the dysbiosis / lack of trace elements
- Regulation-thermography: hot liver values? Deep intestinale values?
- EAV: lack of trace elements / parasite-nosodes / lymph stress /

- Hg / iso propyl alcohol / formol
- Polysan test: Polysan M or COM

PARACELSUS PARASITE THERAPY

Okoubasan Tr. (Sanum)   1st week: every ½ - 1 h., 5-8 dr. under the tongue, starting from 2nd week: 6 x 10 dr., keep under the tongue.

Leptospermum scop. Tinktur (Sanum)
1st +2nd week: every ½-1 h., 5-8 dr. under the tongue, starting from 3d week, 6 x 10 Tr., dr. under the tongue; 6 weeks!

Absinthium of CERIUM   4-6 x 3 drops, lightly diluted, under the tongue; 6 weeks

Diet and detoxification   vegetarian mixed diet, carrot days!

Colon hydrotherapy   1-2 x per week. Liver pack, mustard pack, epsom salt, green tea, manganese, Mapurit Sanum, Selenmethionin

APPENDIX 4A: SIMPLE DIETARY GUIDELINES
FOR THE RELIEF OF THE METABOLISM
AND FOR NEUTRALIZING THE ORGANISM

Dear patient,

We have found it necessary for your body to be generally relieved of stress, the metabolic functions stimulated and the organism as a whole detoxified, thereby stimmulating and improving the regenerative forces of body-tissues, hormonal activity of the glands and esp. the cleansing abilities of the liver and kidneys. The bodies healing forces and immune system are strengthened. A majority of chronic diseases are due to unhealthy eating habits, in particular to too much protein-rich and acid-producing foods.

With the following dietary changes, you make it possible for your body to become, once again, more reactive, the primary condition for each real healing.

The guidance contains only prohibitions. Everything fresh, plant-based, vegetables, fruits, chestnuts, potatoes and leguminous plants are permitted and important, as are cold-pressed vegetable oils. Grains: millet, barley, oats, spelt, wheat-products / bread very reservedly!

- **Little meat: only maximally once per week meat** (better turkey or fish)
- **Absolutely no pork, no sausages** (meat contains many amino-acids and sulfur, is acidic, thickens the body fluids)
- **No milk drinks**
- **Very little cow's milk products / cheese**
- **Absolutely no yogurt, no quark** (cow's milk protein thickens lymph, creates "cold", is builds mucus and burdens the immune system)
- **No sugar and no sugar-containing foods** (sugar is very acid-forming, burdens the metabolism, esp. egg-rich creams, ice cream) honey, pear syrup, maple syrup, cane sugar, etc.: <u>very little</u> sweetner permited
- **No Citrus fruits**
- **Evenings no fruits** (because of fermentation)
- **No fruit juices!** (fruits ferment in the evening, form alcohol, load the liver) (citrus fruits are frequently allergens, much pesticide, acid) <u>little</u> grapefruit juice, or ½ grapefruit permitted to the breakfast
- **No alcohol**
- **Drink large quantities, mineral-poor water** (large quantity of water promotes metabolism, detoxification. 3 litres per day!) Drink esp. between meals, not with meals! (alcohol burdens the liver and decreases its other functions of detoxification).

APPENDIX 4B: SIMPLE DIETARY GUIDELINES
FOR STIMMULATING REGENERATION, DETOXIFICATION AND
NEUTRALIZING ACIDITY

What may and should be regularly eaten?

Grains: In principle, the original grain sorts are very valuable: spelt / millet / oats / barley. Take these daily as flakes, soup, mash, except with proven grain allergy (gluten). Wheat is increasingly problematic and is to be eaten therefore, only little: (bread, conventional grain-flour noodles, etc.!!). The reason lies in modern wheat breeding, which aims at a very high gluten portion (up to 60%). Allergies often develop on gene-technology altered wheat and its flour- preservation products.

Potatoes: Are recommendable, esp. in the evening, as potato soup or baked. Are as nightshade plants, rather "cold".

Vegetables: Are allowed, and should constitute the majority of ones nutrition. Work up to increasing proportions of raw vegetables. Goal: 50% raw vegetables, as salads, etc., esp. sellerie, carrots, radish, avocado, etc.. Particularly good: beans, peas, lentils or also chestnut and avocado! Green vegetables are very mineral- and calcium-rich: salads, broccoli, zucchini, etc.. Tomatoes only few, not raw! (acid, cold !)

Corn: On the cob, polenta, contains important essential amino-acids, minerals.

Fruits: Should represent the bulk of the diet up to noon. Always peel Fruits (pesticides!): apples, pears, seed fruits, as seasonally as possible! Bananas: are very mineral-rich, but produce mucus! Tropical fruits: grapefruit, papaya, pineapple in the morning good, there very enzyme-rich. Otherwise, tropical fruits only in the morning and in small quantity (many people tolerate kiwi and mandarines badly, they often work allergy-strengthening)!

Eggs: Chicken egg (ONLY from organic farms and free-range!!): two to three eggs per week permited: heated up as little as possible: 3-8 min. simmered. No fried eggs or egg-containing baking goods

Rice: As Basmati rice suitably for Allergiker and intestine patients. Whole grain rice would be very mineral, material and vitamine rich, but acidic and digestible with difficulty!

Seed sprouts:
Are very important! Take daily only one type of seed, sprout: cress / soya / alfalfa / wheat sprouts, peas, etc..

Vegetable oils:
Cold pressed, organic: daily 30-50 ml: Flax seed, sunflower, olive oil, ect.

APPENDIX 5: THE REGENERATION OF
THE INTESTINAL FLORA
ACCORDING TO DR. MED. TH. RAU

Terrain therapy
Alkaline-mineral mixtures
Multi-mineral tablets (Burgerstein)

Intestinal mucosa
Mucosa comp. amp. (Heel)
every 2-3 days inject an amp. at M25-point (neural therapy with Procain) or hold for a long time under the tongue and then swallow

Diet according to Dr. med. K. Werthmann
(no milk and milk products, no eggs, no nuts)

Intestinal flora
Beginning: **Fortakehl D5**, 3x1 tabl.
then **Pefrakehl D4 caps.** or drop, 2 weeks
then **Sankombi drops** 2x10 or Mucokehl and Nigersan

Immune stimulation

By chronic infections, infectious tendencies, Colitis, etc.:
By regeneration of the intestinal flora: first one week **Notakehl D5 tabl.** 3x1, then further as above
Utilin and **Recarcin caps.** (Sanum), 1 each per week
Rebas D4 caps. (Sanum CH), 2x1 caps. / day

Dr. Thomas Rau, M.D.
Paracelsus Klinik Lustmühle,
9062 Lustmühle (bei St.Gallen)
Switzerland

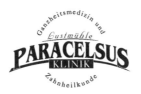

13

The Paracelsus Liver and Gallbladder Detoxification Programme

THE PARACELSUS LIVER CLEANSING CURE / THE PARACELSUS "GALLBLADDER FLUSH"

Short introduction to the topic Liver Cleansing

Apart from our skin, intestines and muscles, the liver is one of the largest organs of the human body. The numerous complex functions of the liver, for example: the direct control of growth and the function of our body cells, the decontamination of blood and lymph and the transformation of nutrients into the bodys own substances (e.g. hormones), are of the greatest importance for good health. Reversly, each malfunctioning of the body, lack of condition or incorrect cell growth, is, at least partly, caused by a bad liver function.

Millions of people in the western world suffer complaints from gallstones. Many people believe that gallstones are found only in the gallbladder. This is a common misunderstanding, because most gallstones are actually found within the liver, where they can form and consolidate themselves from thickened gall, to a gelatin-like, rubbery or even hard consistency. Relatively few appear in the gallbladder, a circumstance which one can determine easily, if one accomplishes the liver cleansing cure.

The therapy is oriented purely on symptoms and does not eliminate the cause of the illness and even prepares, in many cases, the way for still heavier subsequent complaints:

Many adults in the industrialized world – and particularly those, who suffer from chronic diseases, for example: coronary heart illness, arthritis, multiple sklerose, cancer or diabetes – have many to hundreds of gallstones, which clog or even block the gall ducts of their liver. These consist, to the largest part, of clumped gall and cholesterine.

The constant increase of auto-immune illnesses, food incompatibilities, allergies, infectious tendencies (already at an early age) is predominantly a consequence of wrong nutrition and an overloaded defense system. The liver relieves the immune system, by cleaning the blood; it removes both poison materials which result from the body's own metabolism, and those which are introduced from the outside. It expells many toxins into the intestine, eliminates even micro organisms from the blood and produces, beyond that, immune stimulating substances. The liver is the most important filter of our blood, and at the same time, our chemical factory.

The presence of clumps of gall (gallstones) in the liver and gallbladder, substantially disturbs vital processes, like: digestion of food, elimination of waste products and decontamination of harmful substances, which are in the bloodstream.

Gallstones can lead to inflammations in the gallbladder but also to cramp-like contractions of the gallbladder, so-called colic attacks. It is a very common misunderstanding of medicine, that gallstones can only be removed by operation. Our "Gall Cleansing" shows that very frequently, quite large stones can be completely expelled without colic attacks, through the relaxed gall ducts into the intestine. We have already seen single gallstones up to 2cm in diameter! Much more frequently, are however, expulsions of many smaller gallstones, up to 1 cm in diameter!

With the unblocking of the liver gall ducts, the several billione cells of our body can "breath" better again and can receive a sufficient quantity of nutrients; they will be better able to expell waste products and be able to maintain perfect communication with the body's nervous and hormonal systems.

Medicines and diet by Gall Cleansing
The production and flow of gall can be enormously increased with nutrition and plant-based medicines and thus, gall concentrations can be dissolved again.

Dietary guidelines

(see also following "Dietary guidelines for the liver detoxification program")

- Avoid roasted fats, if possible little meat, no butter
- No or very few milk products, no melted cheese
- Lots of vegetables, steamed, raw or very well cooked!
- In the morning, fruits, particularly grapefruit
- Daily, 1 spoon cold pressed, organic, vegetable oil
  (we recommend flax seed-, grape seed-, or olive oil)
- Daily, drink 2–3 litres minerall-poor water, at best warm

Medicines

There are very good, plant based substances for the support of gall function and activation of the liver:

- Absintium (wermut) CERIUM, 3x5 drops
- Taraxacum (dandelion) CERIUM, 3x5 drops
- Carduus marianus (Mariendistel) CERIUM, 3x5 drop
- Winkelmann-Paracelsus Gall tea, 2–3 cups daily
  (contains vervain, celandine, sage, chicory).
- Chelidonium D4, D6, D8 of CERIUM, 3x5 drops
- Mentha piperita (peppermint) CERIUM, 3x5 drops, with cramps, nausea or during hyper-acidity, which frequently accompanies gall problems.

There are also medicines for the dissolution of concentrations of gall, which are even applied in standard medicine and accepted by the health insurance companies. They must be taken, however, on a long-term basis (3–12 months):

- De-Ursil RR (dosage 450 mg/daily for adults)
- Urso Falk (same dosage) active ingredient: Desoxy Cholsaeure

OPTIMAL HEALTH DEPENDS A ON A HEALTHY LIVER

and

A GRAM OF PRECAUTION IS BETTER THAN
A TON OF THERAPY!

DIETARY GUIDELINES FOR THE PARACELSUS LIVER DETOXIFICATION PROGRAM

The exact procedure:
- Begin the morning with a large cup of warm normal water. Water is digested easily and gives the kidney and different body cells the necessary liquid, fast. During the passage of the digestive tract, it rinses waste materials away and activates the "peptic system" of the stomach
- 15 minutes later, you take 2 tablespoons (30 ml) of pure, cold-pressed olive oil, mixed with the same quantity of freshly pressed lemon juice.

For breakfast, you select between:
- 1–2 glass fresh juice: apple, grapefruit, vegetable (carrots, zucchini), grapes, pineapple etc. or
- Green tea (and/or other cleaning herb teas)
- Fresh fruits. Recommendable: peeled and lightly cooked apples. Do avoid however larger quantities of citrus fruits, except ½ grapefruit
- Avocado with fresh lemon juice and olive oil
- Porridge, which must be prepared, however, with water and not with cow's milk, with fresh fruits or berries
- Muesli with raisins and fruits
- No coffee, black tea, sugar!
- No milk and milk products (cheese...)
- no white bread, no wheat products

For **lunch** select between:
- raw or steamed vegetables, always: zucchini, artichokes, carrots, broccoli, red beets, lettuce, sellerie etc. in small quantities: potatoes
- Sprouts: wheat, alfalfa, soja, lentils, among other things.
- Very little whole-meal bread, if it appears necessary to you (spelt...)
- Raw vegetables must always be very finely cut and, just like cooked/steamed vegetables, always with lemon juice and olive oil.

- Intermediate meals: vegetables with lemon juice and olive oil
- ABSOLUTELY PROHIBITED is common salt (sodium chloride). Genuine sea salt and herb spices are permitted

At **dinner,** you should generally eat as little as possible:
- Vegetable juices, green vegetables (e.g. zucchini), carrots, flax seed oil, herb tea
- Steamed spinach and/or other steamed vegetables
- Oats soup
- Finely cut salads with lemon juice and olive oil
- Vegetable soups

Additional therapy measures with the intensive Paracelsus liver-gall cleansing:
- 2x Colon Hydrotherapy with Paracelsus Refloristation (see farther back)
- 2x local hyperthermia over liver and gallbladder
- 2x segmental neural therapy with isopathic-homœopathic remedies over liver and gall, as well as akupunctur point Le3

IMPORTANT

Chew all foods (also the juices and soups) thoroughly – the addition of saliva is enormously important!
Drink much water – between meals, NOT with meals. Do not replace the water with the apple juice, which you get offered within the context of the cure, i.e.: do not drink apple juice against the thirst!

THE LIVER – GALLBLADDER CLEANSE
(according to Nicolaou/Rau)

Preparation

- Drink 1–2 litres apple juice per day for the duration of 6 days. Although we do not recommend these normally, you can also drink the usual apple juice available in stores. Organic apple juice is naturally better. Apple juice works best, in the context of detoxification: it can soften stones and thus facilitate their expulsion from the gall ducts. Due to it's strong effect, it can also lead, in the first days, to a bloated feeling and and/or to thin stool. The fermentation of the juice helps to enlarge the gall ducts. If too many unpleasant reactions arise, then you can dilute the juice with water. Drink the juice slowly, distributed over the day, between meals. Avoid drinking the apple juice directly before or after the meals, or in the late evening.
- The juice is taken additionally to your normal liquid intake. Do not replace this water (against thirst) with apple juice! Follow this Dietary guidelines exactly. Particularly, no animal protein may be eaten during the cleaning phase.
- Begin the cleaning, by drinking or two glass of warm water slowly.
- 15 minutes later, you take 2 tablespoons (30 ml) pure, coldly pressed olive oil, mixed with the same quantity to freshly pressed lemon juice.
- Have breakfast, at the earliest, 30 minutes afterwards.
- If the lemon/olive oil mixture does not agree with you, then eat ripe, sweet peas (on an empty stomach) instead, 30 min. before the breakfast.
- If, after 6 days of the apple juice cure, you feel hungry, you can eat a light breakfast in the morning: cooked grains, fruits or fruit juices.
- No milk or milk products, no animal protein, during the whole cure!!
- At noon: cooked vegetables with rice (however, only with herbs or SOMEWHAT genuine sea salt)

What you can expect:

You will possibly get some soft stool, or diarrhea; whereby, gallstones and food rests will be excreted, perhaps later also together with watery intestinal contents. Look for swimming gallstones in the toilet, these are often at the water surface because of their cholesterine content.

To stones are recogniseable the from their green color, and they have all possible sizes (from pea size to 3 cm) and forms. Large quantities can be expelled at one time in individual cases. Perhaps you can conserve one of the large stones, in order to present it to your family doctor. Be curious as to how you can relieve your body!

THE LIVER-GALL CLEANSE

This instruction refers to the day BEFORE the second colon hydrotherapy

Eat and drink nothing (except water) after 2 PM!

The following schedule is of greatest importance for the success of the cleansing:

6 PM: Mix 4 teaspoons Epsom salts with three cups of water. This quantity is sufficient for altogether four (4) portions: Drink the first portion now. You can take some lemon juice after the first small sips, in order to take the bitter taste in the mouth, or drink the liquid with a straw, so that the taste buds on the tongue are avoided.

8:30 PM: Drink the second ? cup.

9:30 PM: If you have had no bowel movement up to now, make yourself an enema with warm water now. This should release some movement.

9:45 PM: Press one or more grapefruits or lemons. You need about three-quarters of a cup, without fruit pulp. Mix the juice with ? cup olive oil. Add 10 drops walnut-, garlic- or wormwood-tincture. Shake the mixture well, until it is watery. Drink this mixture at approx. 22 o'clock, with frequent urge to bowel movement, somewhat later.

10 PM: Drink the above mixture STANDING, not sitting, however, do not take longer than 5 minutes. Afterwards, lie stretched in bed. This is the simplest way to resease the stones. Lie, the upper body raised with an extra cushion, ABSOLUTLY CALM, for the next 20 minutes. Should you have a nauseas feeling, then you can also lie on the RIGHT side, again with elevated head position, and pull in the knees.
Try to mentally support yourself, by immagining how the stones leave your body. Breathe from the diaphram (= belly breathing).
All this will increase the possibility gall concentrations moving out from

the gall ducts. Do not be concerned by possible colic attack pain: The salts are extending the gall ducts. Try to rest somewhat, or perhaps even to sleep.

If you feel the urge to have a bowel movement at night, then please go to the toilet. Check whether gallstones have already been separated; these are pea-like green or also brownish and swim in the toilet. At night and in the early morning, you might feel "low". This will disappear in the course of the morning.

The following morning, that is, on the day of the second colon hydro-therapy:

6 AM to 6:30 AM: At awaking, but not before 6 o'clock in the morning, you drink the third quarter of the salt solution. If you are very thirsty, you can take warm water BEFORE the salt solution. Remain lying calmly, resting still, possibly meditating. If you feel tired, then lie down again.

8 AM to 8:30 AM: Drink they the fourth and last quarter of the salt solution and rest further.

10 AM to 10:30 AM: Drink a fresh juice of your choice. After a further half hour, eat something fruity. One hour later, you can take a normal, however as light (esp. low in protein and fat) a meal as possible.

Dr. Thomas Rau, M.D.
Paracelsus Klinik Lustmühle,
9062 Lustmühle (bei St.Gallen)
Switzerland

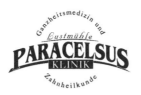

14

Candida – Friend and Helper or "Foe"? New Associations in the Cause of the Candida "Problem"

Yeast fungi on the skin and mucous membranes – Candida – are not only unpleasant and irritating but in numerous cases are the cause of considerable vegetative and neurological disorders as well as diseases of the mucous membranes. Most recently new references have been found concerning the cause of candidiasis in humans: for example, the fact that healthy people with a high level of amalgam are at the same time affected by Candida – though not in a pathogenic but a protective form.

In various investigations and talks, I have shown that not only is Candida a foe which can cause illness for human beings but its natural occurrence is completely justified. Candida must therefore be treated correctly, made less capable of causing disease and not killed.

The pathogenicity of Candida is a sign of the times
In the Paracelsus Klinik we treat numerous patients with vague multiple symptoms. Because of the frequent occurrence of neurological disorders and problems of the mucous membranes which these patients present, traditional medicine would assume them to be under attack from Candida. The investigations which have been carried out are often unsatisfactory: that is, stool tests show false negative results, serology relating to the physical attack is hardly convincing and the symptoms are blurred in such a way that mostly it is assumed that there is a vegetative weakness or a psychosomatic illness. This does the patient an injustice, as the supposedly vegetative and psychological symptoms almost always

improve after a thorough course of milieu therapy and treatment of the pathogenicity of the Candida.

The different methods of diagnosis

Only a small number of analytical methods can prove the presence of Candida:

The best is *darkfield diagnosis* of vital blood: this is not only very important in clarifying the milieu but also extremely useful. It shows the endobiontic attack on a patient, but not that of the Candida on itself. In every case darkfield is of central significance for the biological physician in his/her assessment of the milieu and the proneness to infectious diseases . (However, for the clinical physician it is the clinic which is at the forefront in the assessment of a possible "Candida patient").

EAV *(Electroacupuncture according to Dr. Voll),* the Vega test, Mora testing and kinesiology are suitable only to prove the Candida attack but never suitable for providing evidence relating to pathogenicity.

Thermoregulation diagnosis according to the methods of Professor A. Rost shows only non-specific reactions of the intestinal mucous membrane.

Stool tests are again often of no use: on the basis of several investigations it was possible to confirm that patients who in clinical terms have been indisputably diagnosed as Candida patients can present negative results in stool cultures. This can by explained by the fact that – despite correct methods of transport – Candida culture can die whilst being transported to the laboratory. Proof of this comes from an experiment in which two stool samples from the same patient and the same motion were sent to the laboratory, one by post and the other directly. The findings from the two samples were extremely different. Moreover, in 30% of clinically healthy subjects who presented no Candida symptoms, Candida was found up to a level of 104. And this although no evidence of pathogenicity could be found in the light of the stool cultures. A straightforward attack of Candida is therefore not a disease but a variation. Only in the light of further studies was it possible to prove that all the subjects who were Candida positive yet healthy were exposed to mercury. That means, the Candida cultures in the stools are insignificant and non-specific. Therefore it is absolutely vital to take care that the stool samples are measured while they are still fresh.

Candida serology is very cost-intensive and only shows that Candida is present in the system, but not whether it is pathogenic, so this does not indicate what treatment should be given.

To summarise: based on my own investigations, in every case where Candida is suspected, a DMPS (Dimaval) test (preferably i.v.), *hair mineral analysis* and *darkfield investigations* should be used to check for the patient being exposed to mercury and other heavy metals.

Symptoms

Some of the extremely diverse range of symptoms are shown in the following table. They can be divided into symptoms of the mucous membrane, neurological symptoms and vegetative symptoms:

Exposure to heavy metals and Candida present the same symptoms

Symptoms of the mucous membrane
- Aphthae, chronic sinusitis
- Proneness to infection, throat infections
- Stomach problems, dysbioses
- Colitis, proctitis
- Bronchitis, asthma
- Recurrent cystitis, vaginitis, prostatitis
- Non-articular rheumatism (excess acid)
- Joint problems

Neurological symptoms
- Poor concentration
- Visual disorders
- Headaches, neuralgia
- Paraesthesia, trembling
- Dizziness

Vegetative disorders
- Sweating
- Trembling
- Palpitations
- Interrupted sleep pattern
- Depression
- Emotional disturbance
- Stomach cramps, etc.

You will inevitably find **symptoms of the mucous membrane:** they are the sign of an attack and of dysbiotic modification to the corresponding mucous membranes. The best known are chronic cystitis, vaginitis and prostatitis. Moreover these conditions almost always present a cough which is slightly productive and a whitish livid change in the mucous membrane of the anus and the perianal skin. Very small tears, either in the corners of the mouth or in the folds of the anus, are a frequent occurrence. Stomatitis aphtosa, and in longer attacks Lichen ruber planus too, are both a sign of Candida and of exposure to mercury. Also very typical is chronic sinusitis. Anti-mycotic treatments make the attack worse in the long term, in particular if the cause is not treated (excess acid, exposure to toxins).

Neurological symptoms are both a sign that mycotoxins are being released and possibly also of mistreatment with antimycotics, as mycotoxins and heavy metals are again released by the decomposition of the Candida.

Vegetative disorders can be interpreted on the one hand as a defect of vegetative neuroganglions and mycotoxins, or on the other hand as a localised attack with Candida itself which however until now could not be proven by histological methods. The vegetative and neurological symptoms are however completely identical with those of heavy metal poisoning, which again shows the parallels. These can be explained as follows:

Candida as a form of natural protection
It is well known from Nature that fungi are able to bond with heavy metals. This is even how fungi are used in industrial applications. For

example, in American mines yeast cultures are knowingly introduced into the bore holes. These bond with silver, manganese, gold and other heavy metals so that a large yield can be obtained. In this respect there is a parallel with human beings, as recent investigations show: of about 56 healthy, symptom-free subjects 30 per cent had Candida colonies. Here exceptionally only people with a high level of exposure to amalgam were involved (Hg following DMPS 250 mg i.v. > 100 μg/g of creatinine).

Accordingly, Candida colonisation in humans can be regarded as a natural form of protection of the organism against exposure to heavy metals – the heavy metals are bonded by the Candida and finally excreted. If a fungal attack is treated with chemicals, the fungus is killed and thus at the same time the natural protection against exposure to heavy metals is destroyed. In addition, the toxins which are liberated when the fungus is killed as well as the products of fungal decomposition such as mycotoxins and mercury complexes are released. And Candida – if they are "starved out" or "wiped out" – by a carbohydrate-free diet or by intestinal antimycotics – can change into a protease-forming form, penetrate the wall of the intestine and infiltrate the tissues and circulation in a highly pathogenic form, or they transform themselves into a chronic spore form. This can be seen in darkfield investigations. The treatment of Candida attacks must be therefore be carried out carefully and in particular must start with the milieu.

Fungi must be treated, not killed
Logically the treatment cannot therefore be to kill the fungus itself, but only to change it into the non-pathogenic, protease-forming form. The Sanum preparations made to Professor Enderlein's instructions are suitable for this purpose. For him health is synonymous with a situation in which a balanced milieu exists in the microbial ecology of the human organism and the "balance of symbiosis" is maintained with the help of natural biological control functions. On the other hand Enderlein ascribes illness to the dysbiotic, destructive activity of the endobiontic high valencies which triggers various forms of degenerative diseases, whether degeneration of the cells or degeneration in the sense of neoplasia.

The three stages of treatment

The aims of the treatment of Candida are: first to support the Candida in its role as a detoxifier, secondly to lower its pathogenicity, and thirdly to prevent it filtrating through the intestinal wall into the blood. At the same time the intestinal flora should be built up by using isopathic remedies and a special diet. All this is achieved with the following treatment plan over a period of about a year (the symptoms will begin to improve after 1–4 weeks):

Medications: Initially: one Fortakehl capsule three times daily for two weeks, then one Pefrakehl *(Candida parapsilosis)* capsule or drops (10 drops); at the same time a slow increase with Albicansan drops (beginning with 5 twice daily, then rising to 10 three times daily), from the second week possibly adding Exmykehl suppositories; subsequently for one year Sankombi drops (10 drops) or Mucokehl tablets and Nigersan tablets for the regeneration of high valencies in the cells and systems which enable the Candida to build up.

Diet: The diet should not "starve" the fungus but must build up the wall of the intestine and enable the regeneration of the normal intestinal flora. What is required is a diet which is low in allergens, rich in minerals and is alkaline as laid down by Dr. K. Werthmann and Dr. Thomas Rau. That means, no cow's milk products and eggs, no pork, no citrus fruits and no fruit in the evening (because of fermentation). Industrially-produced sugar in any form, including in drinks, is forbidden. Carbohydrates are permitted, but proteins should be avoided.

Assistance in the removal of heavy metals: The heavy metals (for example, amalgam) are sought out using hair mineral analysis, the Dimaval test and darkfield microscopy and, wherever possible and necessary, removed. Excretion of metal is achieved with Pleo Chelate from Sanum (for adults 15 to 30 drops two to three times daily), with seaweed remedies and Alkala N (1 measuring spoon dissolved in warm water, in the morning on an empty stomach). Colonic irrigation therapy can also help (approximately once every 1–2 weeks, six to eight times in all).

Footnote:

Swiss researchers have for the first time used microorganisms successfully to remove heavy metals from the residue of waste incineration plants.

The fly ash from domestic waste, caught in the filters, contains toxic heavy metals in sometimes considerable concentrations. Now Helmut Brandl's team at the Institute for Plant Biology at the University of Zurich has succeeded in removing a large part of these contaminants from the residue of waste incineration plants with the help of microorganisms. For example, after 24 hours in a bath containing a solution of minute fungi of the *Aspergillus niger* variety, fly ash had lost the following amounts of heavy metals: 81 % cadmium, 66 % zinc, 57 % copper and 52 % lead; also 32 % manganese and 27 % aluminium.

The new technique will make fly ash usable in future as an admixture for building materials which does not damage the environment. Thus two problems have been solved at once: recycling instead of disposal of rubbish – today 70,000 tons of Swiss fly ash are dumped annually as toxic waste, some of it in former mines in Germany – as well as the recovery of the valuable metals contained in the rubbish.

The processes being used at present to clean fly ash require a lot of either energy (until the metals evaporate as they are heated) or chemical solvents (which in themselves are a hazard). On the other hand, with biological leaching using bio-organisms, such disadvantages disappear. (Press release form the Swiss National Fund, September 1996).

Dr. Thomas Rau, M.D.
Paracelsus Klinik Lustmühle,
9062 Lustmühle (bei St.Gallen)
Switzerland

Published in Sanum Post No. 43 1998

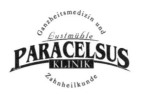

15

Dr. Rau's 7–21 day Fasting Cure

Introduction

Fasting is not Starving – Starving is not Fasting.

During starvation, a person's metabolic activity is considerably reduced and the whole body goes into a "saving mode". During a special kind of Fast, an intensification of the metabolism takes place, along with the massive elimination of poisons, detoxification, and a regeneration and the increased oxidation of the cells and tissue.

The Aim of the Fast

Is to relieve the load on the body's tissues, and to free the body from protein toxins and fatty deposits. At the same time the intestinal flora – a major component of our immune system – and indirectly the whole lymph system, is regenerated.

During the Fast

This is therefore an exceptionally intensive time for the body, rarely leading to weakness. During the fasting time, one can carry out one's work without any problem.

However, it is recommended that a person fasts during a quiet period, for example during a vacation, in order to experience the positive results most intensely. That way one can also carry out the kind of activities that support the fast and the general purification of the body, such as taking showers, light exercising and regular walking.

The second through fourth days are the most difficult. It is during this time that the Fasting Crisis occurs. In other words, this is the point at which the wastes and toxins have loosened but are still circulating inside the body.

The Fasting Crisis can manifest itself through headaches, nausea, shivering, blood pressure disturbances, especially a drop in blood pressure accompanied by fatigue and dizziness. The Fasting Crisis responds best to large quantities of liquid, a hot liver compress or an enema.

Liquids

It is extremely important to drink a large quantity of liquids from the first day onwards. At least three liters a day is recommended. In spite of this, the fast leads to a loss of water in the body and a large part of weight loss is water-related. The actual weight loss amounts to about 2kg of fatty tissue a week.

One should drink half a liter of vegetable juice a day during the fast, best drunk in portions throughout the day. We highly recommend the juices made by Biotta, especially the beet juice, carrot juice or best of all the effervescent juices.

A patient with a sensitive stomach can drink a glass of potato juice once a day.

Half a liter (one bottle) of these vegetable juices should be drunk every day. We recommend that no fruit juice should be taken. We further recommend juices made from organic produce to avoid the additional load of toxins from insecticides and fertilizers.

In addition to the basic quantity of liquid, a drink of 1–2 dl of Alkala N should be taken at 10:00am and 4:00pm: Mix ½ measuring spoon of Alkala N in half a glass of water.

The remaining quantity of liquid (approx. 2 liters) should be taken in the form of tea and of Dr. Rau's Basic Lustmuehler Soup. See the special recipe, which is to be prepared without egg.

We recommend the following teas which favor elimination: Fennel Tea, Wormwood Tea, Nettle Tea, Linden blossom Tea, and Peppermint Tea. These teas should not be sweetened with sugar. We recommend especially a cup of Wormwood Tea daily, as it has a very strong and beneficial effect on Liver-Gall Bladder detoxification.

Food

There are different fasting programs. It is very important to stimulate the digestive juices. In order to do so, ingest only a small quantity of food and chew it very thoroughly and slowly. This should lead to the digestion of proteins which have been stored by the body for many years. Now these can be processed by the gall bladder and intestinal mucous membranes. One must therefore eat only small amounts of food, which will also stimulate the digestive juices: for example, in eating a hard roll and chewing each bite 30 times.

Or take one spoonful of sour milk (buttermilk) or natural Bifidus yogurt or one or two slices of apple etc. In the afternoon one should not eat fruit to avoid fermentation. Instead, eat vegetables or ½ slice of Knackebrot (cracker), or one spoonful of yogurt.

Diet Program

Day 1: The first day is a drainage day and leads to a change in the patient's metabolism.

In the morning, eat raw food or fruit. Be careful of pitted fruit which can easily lead to flatulance.

Day 2: In the morning, drink only tea with a spoonful of honey. It is also recommended to take an enema or colonic during the morning. If this is not possible, we recommend taking Epsom salts in the early morning, which encourages intestinal cleansing.

In the afternoon, take Dr. Rau's Vegetable Broth, if possible however without vegetables (the vegetables are removed and a small amount eaten in the evening).

For lunch, you can eat ½ roll, chewed very slowly so as to be mixed with abundant saliva.

In the afternoon, take another cup of tea and honey, in addition take Alkala N separately (see above).

In the evening, eat the cooked, pureed vegetables or 3 tablespoons of Bifidus Natural Yogurt (no more!)

Days 3–6: In the morning, tea and honey

At lunch, vegetable broth (1–2 pieces of fruit compote can be eaten)

In the afternoon, tea and honey

In the evening, vegetable broth

We recommend another colonic or enema on the 4th–6th days. If that is not possible, then please take Epsom salts daily.

Day 7: Morning, tea and honey

Mid-morning, ½ apple

Lunch, basic vegetable soup (only broth)

Afternoon, apple or corresponding amount of compote

Evening, yogurt (natural Bifidus) and 1 to 2 slices of Knackebrot

The Fast can be repeated once or twice
No symptoms of deficiency should occur with this regime during a period of three weeks. We recommend however the addition of individual homeopathic medicines, which encourage detoxification, plus a combination of vitamins and trace minerals.

Accompanying Medicines
2 x 1 tablet of Cela Multivitamin-Mineral tablets (Burgerstein)

Homeopathic medicines from Heel to encourage drainage of toxins:
Hepar comp.	drink one ampule on day one
Hepeel Amp.	day two
Myosotis Amp.	day three
Muscosa comp. + Ubichinon	day four

In addition, the rebuilding of the intestinal flora is initiated with Fortakehl at 2 x 1 tablet daily. Also, on day 4, Sankombi drops 2 x 10 drops (Sanum) per day.

Subsequent to this Fasting Cure, one should continue with a diet low in animal protein foods for some time. This aids further waste removal and brings the body to a more alkaline condition.

- no pork (including no sausages or cold cuts)
- no sugar or sugary products
- very little dairy products or cheese (initially for 1–2 months, no yogurt or cottage cheese)
- in the morning a lot of fruit, in the evening no fruit
- no wine or cider

In the evening, it is highly recommended to eat a baked potato without cheese, with a little butter or ½ mashed banana. However we do not recommend this during the first week.

Often during the Fasting Cure one must also begin to build up the Immune System and treat other health problems. These can however possibly be prevented through cold showers, exercise, brush massage and the above-mentioned liver wrap.

Fasting is suitable for everyone and leads to a marked stimulation of the system both psychically and physically. It is especially appropriate for rheumatic problems, muscle conditions, chronic illnesses like asthma, tendency to infection, high blood pressure, heart ailments and skin conditions. The cosmetic advantage is considerable. Already after one week the skin is cleaner and tighter, the connective tissue strengthened and the eyes clearer. The accompanying weight loss has already been mentioned above. It is however by no means only overweight people who should fast. Fasting is also healthy for normal or underweight people.

We wish you much success and will be happy to support you during your fast.

Dr. Thomas Rau, M.D.
Paracelsus Klinik Lustmühle,
9062 Lustmühle (bei St.Gallen)
Switzerland

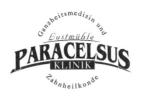

16

Dr. Rau's Intensive Detoxification Diet

EXPLANATION: The diet plan described below is an intensive treatment recommended for those individuals undergoing homeopathic therapy for chronic illnesses, i.e., heavy metal poisoning, tumors or auto-immune disturbances, who want to restore their internal environment to its optimal condition. This diet reduces acidity, has a cleansing effect on the lymphatic system and intercellular substance. In addition, it improves the enzymatic processes which, in turn, influence the metabolic and purification processes. These effects are significantly stronger with this diet in comparison to a normal fasting regimen. However, patients will find that they can maintain a normal level of activity and in fact feel more dynamic and alert as well!

The diet should be maintained for at least *one to three weeks* and can be followed by Dr. Rau's basic diet plan, if desired.

IMPORTANT: *Do not* deviate from this plan. *Do not* eat anything else other than what is indicated in the order it is indicated. Especially, *do not* eat any milk products or meat.

DR. RAU'S DETOXIFICTION DIET PLAN:

BREAKFAST SELECTION	LUNCH SELECTION	DINNER SELECTION
1–2 glasses fresh grapefruit juice	Only raw or steamed vegetables: zucchini, carrots, broccoli, green salad, celery, kohlrabi	Eat as little as possible of the following:
1–2 glasses green tea or Paracelsus "Blutrei-nigungstee" (tea to cleanse the blood)	Cooked, grated potatoes in small amounts	2dl carrot juice or Breusssaft (vegetable juice)
NO COFFEE – NO SUGAR	Bean sprouts: wheat germ, alfalfa soy, chick pea, linseed or lentil	Spinach or other vegetable
1 fresh, peeled apple	Raw vegetables should be grated and prepared with olive oil and lemon juice	Oatmeal soup
½ avocado with lemon and olive oil	**ABSOLUTELY NO SALT**	2 x per week, one soft boiled organic egg
A small amount of porridge	A grapefruit as dessert	Finely grated celery root-, potato-, or cucumber salad with olive oil and lemon juice
NO WHEAT PRODUCTS		
NO MILK PRODUCTS		**CHEW ALL YOUR FOOD WELL!**

BETWEEN MEALS: In the morning: ½ an apple, peeled, some dried fruit, or 2–3 nuts. Otherwise: ½ raw carrot, be sure to chew this well; 2 dl. apple juice or lemon juice; **Dr. Rau's Basesuppe; Löwenzahntee. DRINK LOTS OF WATER!** The total amount of fluids you should be taking in between meals should be at least 2–3 liters!

FURTHER INFORMATION AND ADDITIONAL THERAPIES:

THE "GALLBLADDER FLUSH" (NICOLAOU AND BOWMAN):

You can intensify the cleansing of the gallbladder by doing the following:

- During the first three days of this diet by drinking 30 ml of olive oil in 30 ml of fresh squeezed, organic lemon juice in addition to the recommended intake.

- On the third day, take 15–20 grams of EPSON SALT in a glass of warm water. (Note: The taste is quite bitter/salty, have a glass of plain water nearby). This acts as a laxative.

- On the fourth day, continue with the olive oil 30ml and lemon juice 30ml, however, **DO NOT EAT AFTER LUNCH!** Instead, take another 20 grams of EPSON SALT in a glass of warm water (as above). Drink plenty of **Löwenzahntee** or Paracelsus *"Darmtee"* (tea for the intestinal tract).

- In addition: 6 x 15 drops **OKUBASAN;** 3 x 5 drops **ABSINTHI-UM CERES** should be taken the entire week.

You will have a considerable amount of diarrhea, which will subside within a few hours. This is the intensive purification of the gallbladder in which gall stones can also be effectively passed and eliminated. (Observe the character of the stool).

Carrot juice, olive oil, apple juice and lemon juice are all gallbladder stimulants that aid in purifying the gallbladder. In addition, carrot juice and raw carrots eliminate parasites. It would be advantageous to include all of the above mentioned juices and olive oil in your routine daily diet.

COLON-HYDROTHERAPY: Also referred to as HIGH COLONIC ENEMA. This is advantageous along with the purification diet since this is actually a bathing of the large colon. If possible, it should be done 1–2 times. If you are also doing the gallbladder flush regimen, it is a good idea to do this *before the first day* and *after the fourth day.* (See accompanying material).

COFFEE ENEMA: This is a simple yet very effective treatment you can do easily on your own at home. It activates the liver and promotes the detoxification of this organ as well. (See accompanying material).

Dr. Thomas Rau, M.D.
Paracelsus Klinik Lustmühle,
9062 Lustmühle (bei St.Gallen)
Switzerland

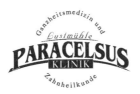

17

Using Biological Regulation Therapy for Inflammatory-Rheumatic Diseases

The chronic inflammatory and chronic exudative diseases of the mucous membranes are amenable to conventional medical treatment usually only via anti-inflammatory and/or immunosuppressive means. These diseases in particular – chronic inflammatory joint diseases, rheumatoid arthritis, intestinal (colitis), bronchial (asthma) – are known for their stubborn resistance to conventional medical therapy. The high rate of recurrence after therapy is cut back is likewise well known. From a biological-regulative point of view, this is quite understandable, since the mucous membrane organs, with their enormous surface areas, are vital regulatory and eliminatory organs, whose oversecretion when disturbed corresponds to a need of the organism's. This excretion is purifying and detoxifying, and thus constitutes a regulatory function in the interest of the body as a whole.

When, therefore, the holisically-orientated physician views the mucous membrane "diseases" not as diseases in and of themselves, nor as terminal states, but rather as goal orientated regulatory processes, then not only does the whole process make more sense , but so do the diagnostic and therapeutic measures. From the regulatory-medical viewpoint, mucous inflammations are there for regional or general elimination in the service of detoxification, and can only be suppressed for short periods of time. The toxic substances – the disturbing agents – must be found and channelled out.

The mucous membrane organs are the body's most powerful regulatory organs, and they react to "foreigners" with their own unique exudation to stimuli throughout the body. When suppressive therapy is used, the result is often remote secondary disease, since in these cases the necessary elimination has not taken place and the toxic agent is now stored elsewhere, doing its harm there. Thus, amyloidosis can follow polyarthritis or colon cancer can succeed colitis.

The mucous membrane organs make up a functional "detox" unit – which explains the ability of chronic diseases to migrate to other mucous membrane organs. Thus, the asthma sufferer can get arthritis, or colitis will lead to colitis-arthritis. The "burned-out" condition of a mucous membrane disease in older patients is mostly prognostically poor, with damage to fundamental cellular functions being expressed in a cellular-degenerative or even neoplastic stage of disease.

The clinical picture of polyarthritis

With the background presented here, the diagnosis and treatment of polyarthritis, taken as a sample disease, can be seen with particular clarity. The following descriptions are based on years of treatment cycles for this syndrome. In addition, over 20 arthritis patients were kept under observation for more than two years. All patients had already had more than two years of anti-inflammatories and had undergone basic therapy with Gold/d Penicillamin-/Resochine or Immurek.

At the beginning of therapy, all patients had severe polyarticular symptoms accompanied by swelling. Most of the patients were seropositive – i.e. positive with rheumatoid factor – or had elevated ANAK. Two patients were diagnosed with Bechterew's Disease, two children had juvenile arthritis and the rest of the patients had chronic polyarthritis. Results of the therapy: for over 70% of the patients, their condition was improved, in some cases totally healed, despite reduction of the immunosuppressives and Cortisone and despite, in most cases, reduction or even discontinuation of antirheumatics. Besides the subjective findings, the objective parameters (BSR, ANAK, swelling) confirmed this well.

The causes and initiators of the disease

The diagnosis and the subsequent therapy must always be highly individualized and broad-based. The "purpose" of the mucous membrane reaction must be sought. The patient's constitution and disposition must here also be recognised and bound into all therapeutic considerations. In their function as vital eliminatory organs, the overtaxed mucous membranes must be relieved by stimulating other eliminatory systems (intestines, kidneys, skin, lungs). The intestines must above all be included in any and all treatment.

There are various causes and initiators for arthritis that need to be considered (Table 1). Some clari-fications are in order here to promote an understanding of the course the diagnostic process takes. Our experience has shown that chronic arthritis is

CAUSES AND INITIATORS OF ARTHRITIS

- Food allergies
- Elevated arachidonic acid / excess protein
- Foci of disturbance
- Acid-base balance
- Antioxidant deficiency
- Trace element deficiency
- Toxic stress

Table 1

very often associated with food intolerances. This can be seen very clearly in typical regulatory thermography findings. An important indicator of this is the often strikingly positive response of joint ailments to a hypoallergenic diet á la Werthmann (Table 2), which we have slightly modified for our purposes. (Table 3).

Food allergy shows up in a patient history most typically in the form of earlier susceptibilities to infection, in various allergies and skin problems and immune system disturbances induced by exhaustion or over-burdening of the Peyer's Patches in the small intestine. Regulatory thermography depicts the typical findings of a hyperregulating small intestine, with low values over the appendix and small intestine, hot abdominal lymph regions and often with over-taxed (low) stomach values; subsequent readings show still-blocked thymus values.

Other indicative methods are also possible and usable, but often only indicate secondary allergies, to specific foods, for example. Most of the time, proteins in cow's milk and its products represent the fundamental allergen. In this context, exposure in early infancy is decisive, during which the child was not fully suckled by its mother for at least six or more months.

Further important pathogenic factors

The most frequent inflammatory joint disease is chronic polyarthritis co-caused by a dysregulation of the immune system. The inflamed articular process is determined by the amount of type 2 prostaglandins which develop from arachidonic acid (Eicosanoids) (Table 4). Since it is an unsaturated fatty acid, arachidonic acid is introduced to the organism exclusively through animal fats

---

IIYPOALLERGENIC DIET
á la Dr. K. Werthmann

no **Cow's milk / Milk Products**	*no* **Fruits in the Evening**
	no sweets or sweet drinks
no **Hen's Eggs / Egg Products**	fish or meat twice a *week* at most drink lots of liquids
no **Pork, Ham, Bacon,** sardines, kippers, rabbit	and vegetable juices
	Table 2
no **Citrus Fruits,** Kiwi, etc.	

---

in the diet. Not only do the inflammation-inducing prostaglandins derive from arachidonic acid, so do the Leucotrienes, which have a suppressive effect on the immune system and the macrophages; added to which, thromboxanes are also produced, with their aggregation effect on thrombocytes, and histamines as the effectors of allergic ailments.

Thus, one can understand why a diet free of animal fat and protein improves all these diseases. But, along with the elimination (or at least reduction) of arachidonic acid, the synthesis of type 1 prostaglandins by means of trace elements and antioxidants must be promoted. For this purpose, the introduction of high doses of evening primrose oil is thera-peutically indicated.

BASIC SOUP á la DR. THOMAS RAU
(rich in basic substances and minerals)

Preparation
- Celery
- Green beans or lentils
- Zucchini equal portions, cut up fine
- Low boil for 15 minutes, then remove vegetables
- Broth can be seasoned with Nahrin Bouillon, vegetarian, (no meat bouillon, no salt)

The soup is best eaten on the same day, but no later than the next day.

Table 3

It has been shown in comprehensive studies that fasting reduces the inflammatory para-meters considerably, and that a strict vegetarian diet effectively lowers the arachidonic acid level. Thus, diet is an important factor in the treatment of rheumatic dis-eases. Cortisone and non-steroidal antirheumatics inhibit the synthesis of both kinds of prostaglandins and lead to a build up of arachidonic acid, thereby favouring a recur-rence of the disease after these substances are discontinued. If they are to be used at all, they should always be combined with large doses of evening primrose oil and antioxidants.

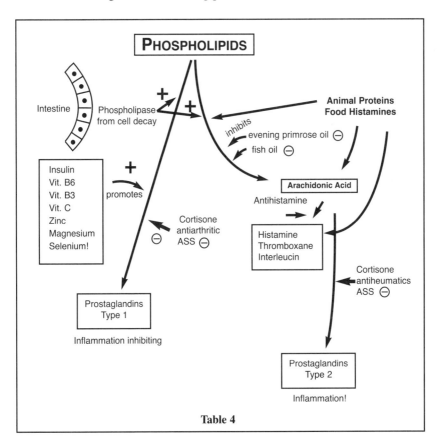

Table 4

The great influence of foci of disturbance in the body

Disturbance foci in the body, representing – not just in the form of abscessed teeth – harmful factors, and being pathological (often bacterially) previously damaged tissues, alter the basic mesenchymal function. Thus, they can trigger or

TONSIL MIX
• *Penicillium chrysogenum*   amp.
• Peyer's Patches extract 4X   amp.
• Tonsilla comp
• Licocaine 1% 5ml
Plus *possibly* – tonsillitis nosode
– citric acid amp.
Table 5

exacerbate any chronic ailment. Often, though, additional factors are first necessary, which explains how a disturbance focus can remain "mute" for years. Disturbance foci are quite frequently the initiators of rheumatic disease. Regulatory thermography turns up disturbance foci in over 70% of chronic illnesses. Our experience shows that over 50% of the rheumatic patients treated by us were improved merely by the introduction of disturbance field therapy.

We implement disturbance field therapy along the lines of Huneke's neural therapy. But, especially for foci in and around the teeth, we almost always add *Penicillium chrysogenum* 7X to the Lidocaine, since these foci often involve old fused bacterial residues – often on gram-positive pathogens – for which *Penicillium chrysogenum* is the agent of choice. About 80% of the disturbance foci are situated in the regions teeth/jaw/sinuses/large intestine. By the way, it's worth mentioning that abnormal bacterial colonizations of the paranasal sinuses can act as disturbance foci themselves, and can thus have enormous disturbing influence on the large intestine. We therefore prescribe, for every chronic patient, intermittent regulatory therapy for the paranasal sinuses, consisting of nose drops containing *Candida parapsilosis*, *Penicillium chrysogenum* and *Mucor racemosus* + *Aspergillus niger*, 2-3 drops taken 4 times daily.

For us, a sorting-out of the disturbance foci by means of regulatory therapy and pantomographic x-ray examination prior to the actual start of treatment belongs to our total therapeutic concept. Intestinal cleansing, usually with enemas or colon hydrotherapy, are also part of it. In the process, any disturbance foci that might be present are detected and noted anamnestically and neural-therapeutically. Disturbance-focus-induced polyarthritis responds especially well to this therapy. A compound injection that has proven itself in disturbance focus therapy is the one we call "Tonsil Mix" (Table 5)

A number of cases have taught us that, when basic therapy and diversion fails, further disturbance foci must be thoroughly and intensively sought out. Not infrequently, multiple disturbance foci are responsible. We emphatically recommend sanitation (which means, as a rule, extraction) of all root-canaled, dead and impacted teeth. This applies above all to the first and second teeth, but as well to the molars (which have a relationship to the large intestine in Voll/Volkmer's schema), which are often disturbance sources due to their focal character.

The influence of the acid-base balance

Investigations of most rheumatic patients indicate depleted acid buffers (bicarbonate/alkali reserves) and elevated acid elimination via urine, stool, skin and stomach. As we know acids are produced as a result of cell metabolism with

---

THE CLARIFICATION PROCESS

Patient history	Dietary
	Stanching / Susceptibility to Infection / Tonsils /
	Operations / Eczema Atopy
Physical appearance	Scars / Teeth / Physique / Congestions
	Type / Constitution, Iris Meridians
Laboratory	– BSR Hb, Lc, Thc, HK
	– ANAK, AST
	– Uric acid, Total Proteins
	– Stool Candida

Table 6

---

vesicular breathing, but they are also introduced by an acid excess in their diet and water. A not insignificant share also arises by way of lactate formation in blocked mitochondrial vesicular breathing and anaerobic energy exchange. This is a well-known significant cancer-causing factor. In an over-acidic situation the body attempts to eliminate these acid equivalents (mostly as proteins) through the mucous membranes. This can generate pathological conditions in all mucous membrane organs and then cause disturbance, in the form of protein complex deposits, of the mesenchyme and connective tissue.

Therefore, re-equilibrating an acid-base balance that has swung over to the acid side is indispensable for all rheumatic patients. This is achieved by a direct supply of bases as well as increased binding of acids to minerals, without neglecting the excretion of acids by all possible avenues. The measures constituting effective treatment include an adapted diet, alkaline supply via

---

What answers are given by

REGULATORY THERMOGRAPHY

- General regulatory ability
- Homeopathically treatable?
- *Disturbance sites?* Blockages?
- Malignant terrain?
- Food allergy?

Table 7

SPECIAL EXAMINATIONS

- *Pantomogram x-ray*
- *Thermography*
- *Darkfield microscopy*
- Hair mineral analysis
- Full acupuncture (opt.)
- Dimaval Test (opt.)

Table 8

---

appropriate minerals – especially recommended in this context is an Alkala-infusion and an improvement of the citric acid cycle.

About antioxidant and trace element deficiencies

Because of high environmental pollution, as well as existing metabolic deficits in vitamins and enzymes, the body's antioxidative defense mechanisms may no longer adequately fulfil their protective functions. This ultimately leads to cell damage throughout the organism, since the cytotoxic substances and free radicals remain active in the body. Therefore, cellular metabolism and the functions of the detoxifying eliminatory organs are scaled down, so that the toxic substances they take up are no longer adequately metabolized and rendered harmless. Consequently, reactive substances build up in the organism, especially in the interstices, but in the joints as well, where oxidative processes can cause excess phagocytosis and lytic damage to cartilage and collagen. This is why a good supply of antioxidants and catalysts of cell respiration is an important component of rheumatic therapy, as it is of any treatment of degenerative diseases.

The process of comprehensive clarification

The clinical history offers the first indications as to possible disturbance foci and dietary allergies for the necessary comprehensive clarification prior to beginning treatment (see Tables 6-10). Determining the patient's constitutional state, the milieu and the general reaction pattern is also of great significance, in this phase of the examination. To the dietetic and medical measures to be taken later. Evaluating the reaction pattern is done by additive methods. The irises, for example, can point to degenerative or congestive tendencies. Physiognomy and physical appearance also indicate dispositions. From the totality of clarifications one then derives the consequences for the steps and measures of a biological course of treatment (Table 10).

Regulatory thermography (mentioned above) is very helpful in determining the organism's reactive capability and in seeking out disturbance fields, as is darkfield microscopy for detecting excess protein or endobiont infestation and as an indication of the state of cellular breathing. Darkfield microscopy also gives an indication as to the need for diversion measures as well as isopathic and/or immunological medications. In darkfield microscopy of chronic inflammatory diseases, enormous findings of reduced resistance and pathological intra- and extracellular developmental forms of certain microorganisms often manifest themselves. In these cases, a longer-term treatment of the patient with isopathic medications is part of the basic rheumatic therapy. The relevant biological preparations, in all their forms of administration, come to the fore in any such drug treatment.

The choice of means depends of course on the type of affliction and disease, but also on the nature and disposition of the patient, of whom may represent the "Mucor" type. The "tubercular" patient, on the other hand, requires preparations corresponding to *Aspergillus niger*, such as *Mycobacterium phlei* and *Bacillus cereus* – but also heat and catalysts. The "congestive" type tends to an excess of yang and, as a metabolic patient, needs primarily *Mucor racemosus*, *Bacillus*

DARKFIELD MICROSCOPY

In Clinical Practice:
- Milieu?
- Excess protein?
- Immune system activity
- Protites?
- leukocyte motility?
- Endobiont infestation?
- Cell resistance? / Vesicular breathing?
- => EMPHASIS in the treatment
- Diversion?
- Protein reduction?
- Endobiont treatment?
- Immune system stimulation?

Table 9

CONCLUSIONS DRAWN FROM CLARIFICATIONS FOR BIOLOGICAL THERAPY

=> Individual therapy<=
=> Causative therapy (opt)<=

- Food allergy?   – milk
    – animal protein
    – histamine

- Diversion crucial?   – colon hydro.
    – *fasting*

- Acid – base therapy?

- Disturbance field purification necessary?
    – teeth
    – head
    – intestines

- Energetic / immune system "build-up" crucial?

- Detoxification   – catalysts
    – ozone
- Substitution therapy necessary?

Table 10

subtilis, Alkala, diversions, diet and, if needs be, fasting. In some cases, a hair mineral analysis is undertaken as a supplementary investigation into patient stress, which yields indications of possible chronic toxic stresses – as, for example, heavy metals – as well as of long-term hyperacidity.

Basic therapy is "multifactorial"

Any therapy which has to date been used successfully on rheumatic patients is always "multitrack" and "multi-factorial" (Tables 11 and 12). If intestinal cleansing, base therapy and diversion are strictly adhered to and correctly carried out, then the anti-inflammatory can quickly be reduced and precipitated. The multitrack aspect of the treatment also encompasses the important immune system organ, Peyer's Patches, since they are usually affected in polyarthritis cases because of reduced performance. To counteract this, patients receive, over a 1-3 month period, one capsule 2-3 times daily of Rebas 4X (Peyer's Patches extract).

As a rule, isopathic therapy with fungal preparations must be carried out long-term, i.e. a year or more. With joint involvement and synovial problems, *Mucor racemosus* in tablet form must above all be given; for older patients, it is recommended that the dosage start low and be raised gradually in ex-pectation of a Chondrite accumulation at the outset. Diversion treatment is indispensable in this context, including *Mucor racemosus* diversion at one ampule per week. The administration of *Mucor racemosus* can also be combined with lactic or citric acid.

Not infrequently, there exists in patients a bacterial stage for which the administration of *Penicillium chrysogenum* is recommended in the first 2-3 weeks of treatment. This proven preparation is often administered periodically, intra-articulary and combined with Lidocaine. Any other acute illness of the arthritic patient should be treated with *Penicillium chrysogenum*, 2-3 tablets daily, and roughly during a week in which the *Mucor racemosus* treatment is to be interrupted.

BIOLOGICAL ARTHRITIS THERAPY

Always "multitrack"!!

- *Acid-base / Intestines*
- *Basic therapy!*
  (–>Table 12)
- Individual according to *special clarifications*
  – disturbance foci
  – diversion
  – food allergy

Table 11

Last but not least among the preparations we've discussed is *Aspergillus niger*, which is always recommended when there is a collagen problem which finds its expression in rheumatic complaints in ligaments, vertebrae, bones and as Bechterew's disease. In these cases, 2 tablets daily are administered. If an intracellular infestation with high endobiont stages exists, then the *Aspergillus niger* is always given together with *Mucor racemosus*. The *Aspergillus niger* Chrondrite evidently favours the passage of the endobionts through the cell walls.

Summary and conclusion

Chronic polyarthritis is not a hermetically isolated disease unit, but rather an outcome of many pathological factors. It responds quite well to biological regulatory therapy if it is applied on a broad front. Among the cases we have treated, we have been able to achieve clear improvement in over 80% of the cases, as regards both arthritic activity and other symptoms as well. Regulatory treatments are not in competition with conventional medical therapies, but after a while do make them dispensable. Very important to a total therapy of chronic

"BASIC" THERAPY FOR
INFLAMMATORY RHEUMATIC DISEASES

1.   De-Acidification   >> = Obligatory!

>> • Diet animal proteins, basic soup, sugar

>> • Minerals: magnesium/calcium 2 x 250-500 mg

>> • **Base supply** *Alkala N*

   • Lactic acid

   • (folic acid 15-30 mg/ day)

2.   Alteration /Immune System "Stimulation"

   • Intestinal Cleansing

   • Citric acid

   • Quinone (Heel)

>> • Peyer's Patches extract 4X 3 x 1 -> 2 x 1 for months!

>> • Utilin strong, 1 capsule/week

   • *Bacillus firmus* strong, 1 capsule/week

   • *Bacillus cereus* strong, 1 capsule/week

   • Cupping, segmental neural therapy, etc

>> • *Fasting, Werthmann Diet*

3.   Milieu Therapy

   • Begin with : *Penicillium chrysogenum* 5X 2-5 tablets once a day

>> • Then *Mucor racemosus* or *Mucor racemosus /*
     Aspergillus niger for one year!

4.   Substitution

   A Antioxidants -> INHIBIT INFLAMMATION

>> ⎧ Vitamin E   500-1500 IU/day
   ⎪ Vitamin C   1-3g/day
   ⎨ DL-methionine
   ⎪ Selenium   50-200µg
   ⎪ Zinc   20-50mg 3 tid
   ⎩ Manganese

>> EVENING PRIMROSE OIL   2-4 grams/day

   B Pain Therapy
   Vitamin B6   100-300mg/day
   Magnesium orotate   250-500 mg 3 tid
   Wobenzyme
   Vitamin E
   DL-methionine

>> Alcohol, Nicotine   Forbidden!
   Histamine stop
   (DL-phenylalanine   750 mg 3 tid)

Table 12

polyarthritis are the fol-lowing therapy factors: diversion, milieu therapy using isopathic medications, trace element supple-ments and the administration of antioxidants.

Dr. Thomas Rau, M.D.
Paracelsus Klinik Lustmühle,
9062 Lustmühle (bei St.Gallen)
Switzerland

Published in Explore! Volume 6 Number 5 1995

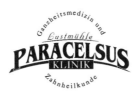

18

Biological Regulation Therapy in Cases of Intestinal Disease, Focusing on Diverticulitis and Recurrent Colitis

The intestine, in particular the colon, with the enormous surface of its mucous membrane measuring up to 1200 m2, is a centre for the body's regulatory processes. The intestine also has enormous vitality as a result of its ability to renew and reconstruct itself very quickly in only a few days, and this vitality can express itself very intensely in symptoms. These symptoms, whether (for example) diarrhoea, flatulence or even painful inflammatory reactions, bring the patient to the doctor's door.

However, these symptoms are not a disease in themselves but the expression of intense regulatory processes, and their message regarding the whole of the body must be recognised and supported. Merely suppressing the symptoms through the use of medications – that is, without removing the cause of the regulatory processes causing the symptoms – will lead to an actual disease of the intestine or immune system: for example, as the result of long-term antiexudative or anti-inflammatory therapy. In such cases the intestine and the Peyer's patches which are found in it can be permanently damaged by the deposition of toxic substances or excessive, long-term strain on the immune system when there is intolerance towards certain foodstuffs; enterohepatic toxicity may also occur.

Thus it is understandable that in what follows the treatment of diverticulitis is very similar to that of ulcerative colitis or Crohn's disease. These therapies are primarily the support and stimulation of excretion, the avoidance of all allergenic substances in food and the stimulation of the regulatory functions of the intestine. The intestine often blocks allopathic therapy in many different ways because of its extremely high level of vitality, on the other hand it is very open to regulatory biological therapy.

Experiences of therapy from the practice

In our general medical practice and in healing medicine, over a period of more than two years we observed and treated over 30 patients with clinically typical diverticulitis and recurrent colitis. These patients were given a course of empiric regulatory therapy, including a special diet and detoxification therapy. The following criteria were used as the basis of this therapy:

- The patient had suffered at least one relapse
- There were pains in the abdomen which were strong, constant or cramp-like in a particular region, lasting at least one day
- There was localised peritonism
- There were disorders of the stool regulation mechanism which were acute and/or were recorded in the patient's medical history.
- A limit of approx. 12,000/mm3 had been reached for the number of leukocytes.

According to most patients' medical history, shortly before the relapse being treated there had been a period of less attention to diet (as around holiday periods) with increased consumption of protein, frequently combined with an increase in the consumption of foods containing sugar and long periods of sitting. In most patients the episode being treated was already the nth relapse. When asked, all patients complained of troublesome stinking flatulence over a long period which showed decomposition of the intestinal flora and/or dysbiosis. More than half the patients had already suffered from episodes of haemorrhoids, and all the patients had already had yellowish paste-like deposits on the back of the tongue for a long period, thus already showing signs of intestinal hepatic overload. The average age of all the patients was only 54 years, and the number of people of each sex was almost exactly equal.

Ten patients had already undergone a coloscopy on one occasion, and all the patients had previously been treated with antibiotics or even as hospital in-patients because of diverticulitis or episodes of colitis. Almost all the patients had already been given a source of laxatives. It appeared that none of the patients that we observed had previously been informed about the connections between foodstuffs which cause decomposition, foods which contain sugar and therefore promote the growth of fungi, and the dysbiosis which is the root cause of diverticulitis, i.e. insufficiency of the intestinal flora. Again and again in our healing centre we saw post-operative patients who had undergone sigmoid resections, who before their attack and afterwards had never been treated consistently with a special diet and/or by building up the the symbiotic flora.

Results of examinations showed chronic conditions

The results of examinations always showed strong pain in the region subjected to pressure, localised peritonism, in the majority of cases on the left side. The patients were slightly to moderately adipose, with a flabby abdomen and weak stomach muscles, and generally did not practise abdominal breathing. Several patients were already showing signs of a big reduction in intestinal sounds in certain regions: this was a bad sign and showed that there had been a transition from the reaction and excretion phase into a deposition phase according to Reckeweg. Two patients had already got a hard diverticular tumour, and one had even got an inflamed stenosis through which it was hardly possible to pass the single use catheter. However, after approximately 2 weeks' treatment this could no longer be detected in control colonoscopy.

Laboratory investigations are not generally very productive and hardly help the medical practitioner to make good decisions about treatment. Even during episodes of strong pain the BSR values could be normal; these are probably more strongly linked to hepatic reaction, the protein situation and enterohepatic autointoxication. The IC values were sometimes raised, sometimes normal, did not correlate with the strength of the clinical picture and in individual cases could be used in neither diagnosis nor therapy.

The stool tests for occult blood were only partially positive and also could hardly be used for decisions on therapy; however, they were important for the diagnostic strategy in that all the patients with a positive haemoccult result had a colonoscopy after the acute phase. One cancerous adenoma of the intestinal villi was found, and we were able to operate and remove this. After the pain had subsided and following treatment, in almost all patients the haemoccult tests were again for the most part negative.

In cases of diverticulitis/colitis, the stool bacteriologies show an increase in candida levels, which is a very important indication of dysbiosis. This is also described by Kolb (with candida levels of up to 80% in cases of colitis) and *Werthmann/Hartmann* in Sanum Post no. 19. Candida infection is always pathological, but it cannot easily be tested for, and unfortunately it is usually not tested for in stool bacteriologies and is even normally interpreted only as a "super-infection". To prove its presence a fresh stool is required: it may not be more than one day old at the time of the test. Infection with candida always requires treatment and is usually a long-term condition. In 80% of tests on diverticulitis patients we have been able to prove the growth of candida, whilst other authors found it occurring in only 5% of people with healthy intestines.

The CEA titres in serum cannot be used as aids to decisions in diagnosis or therapy: they showed unstable results scattered over a large area. However, we consider that CEA values in serum of above 5 ng/ml should be re-checked, also where haemoccult results are found to be positive at the same time, indicating the need for colonoscopy – which, however, is only carried out when the acute diverticulitis episode has subsided as a result of the course of treatment which I am about to explain.

Before therapy commenced, the results of the stool tests were almost without exception on the acid side, probably as a sign of acid fermentation or an "emergency outlet" for intestinal elimination of acid. The pH value of the stools of people with healthy intestines and those whose acid-base metabolism is balanced is alkaline. In a similar manner to the findings of previous antibiotic therapies, the acid milieu also favours candida life-cycles and thus provides ideal conditions for enteral fungal infections.

Important aspects of the therapy

The holistic treatment of diverticulitis, which is also very similar to that for other forms of colitis, even Crohn's disease and ulcerative colitis, always has to be carried out very closely and on a very individual basis because of the acuteness and gravity of the illness. Essentially it achieves:

- Cleansing of the intestine and excretion of toxic products
- Building up of the intestinal flora
- Regulation of the pH value
- Building up of the immune system

To do this the therapy consists of an adjustment to the diet, enemas, control of symbiosis with Sanum remedies, an extra supply of alkalis, replacement of minerals and stimulation of the immunobiological system with Sanum remedies.

DETAILS OF THE TREATMENT

The medicinal diet

There are many publications on diet in cases of colitis, e.g. by *Waerland, Schaub, Rauch (according to F.X.Meyer),* which are highly recommended as reading matter. To these results I should essentially only like to add the criterion of hypoallergenicity, taking into consideration the enormous increase in food allergies and other forms of reaction against food, particularly to animal protein. This does not only include meat but also cow's milk and hens' eggs. This is described fully in the book *"Enterale Allergien"* (Enteral allergies) by Werthmann.

Our diet for the course of treatment consists of the following:

1. Restriction of food intake for 2 to 3 days to relieve pressure on the intestine and to clear it of protein. If the haematocrit values are above 40%, the patient can fast for a longer period. During this phase the patient takes only herb teas, 1 to 2 litres per day, in the form of very weak camomile, peppermint or fennel tea, together with approximately 0.5 litres of Breuss juices.

2. Then follows a slow building up with a basic soup made up as follows: celery/celeriac, green beans, instead of beans possibly lentils or potatoes and courgettes. Chop everything up quite finely into even-sized pieces and cook gently for 10 to 20 minutes. Then strain off the vegetables and serve only the vegetable broth: 300 - 500 mls each morning, to be drunk one sip at a time.

3. According to how the pain is continuing or reducing, after 3 to 6 days the patient is given mashed potato, carrot soup, possibly hard rolls which should be chewed until they are well mixed with saliva, or – with care – sour milk products, also gruel, etc.

4. After this, the food intake is slowly built up again, always with the emphasis on alkaline foods and with a complete ban on meat (at least in the beginning), and to accompany this at least Alkala N should be prescribed.

5. After about one week raw food is added which is retained for longer, particularly very finely grated carrots which as a result of their high beta-carotene content have an anti-inflammatory and anti-oxidative effect which prevents against carcinomas.

6. There is a permanent ban on all pork products in view of the allergens contained therein, the histamine and because of the adrenalin-type substances in meat; the ban also helps to reduce the decomposition of the flora.

7. There is a complete and permanent ban on industrially-produced sugar and all foods containing sugar, in order to achieve a reduction in the candida flora which are always pathological and which in cases of diverticulitis are for the most part chronic.

8. In the long term we recommend a hypoallergenic diet (according to Werthmann, slightly modified) which does not include any cow's milk and milk products, no hen's eggs and egg products, no pork, no sardines or anchovies, no rabbit meat, no citrus fruits or kiwis and no food or

drinks which contain sugar. This diet is continued in the long term because colitis, like diverticulitis, is mostly the expression of a disorder of the body's ability to regulate itself which has happened a long time in the past, resulting in strain on and depletion of the intestinal immune system. During the period of rebuilding the intestinal flora and the villi of the mucous membrane, these should be confronted as little as possible with substances known to be most frequently allergenic, and so this particular diet is to be recommended in the majority of chronic diseases where the immune system is under strain and where there is inflammation. In the regulation therapy which we carry out, we very frequently find allergies to foodstuffs in all types of regulation disorders and diseases, and this justifies this diet over and over again.

9. In the long term we recommend a high proportion of raw foods in the diet with finely grated vegetables, but a slow and careful increase in the amount of raw food is indicated. In order to avoid unrest at night right from the beginning, the patient should avoid eating raw foods in the evening. The action of the beta-carotene in raw food, which protects the mucous membrane, is important. Here we can also assume that it will prevent carcinomas, which is particularly important in cases of diverticulitis with its enormously increased incidence of colon cancer. The high proportion of plant fibres in raw foods also helps to prevent the formation of toxic products which lead to decomposition – such as carcinogenic nitrosamine, in particular.

10. The very common lack of magnesium, particularly in colitis patients, makes the colitis worse with bowel spasms and more diarrhoea. Care should therefore be taken to supplement the diet with sufficient magnesium, particularly as magnesium works as an alkali and bonds with acids from the metabolism of protein. As a medication magnesium is best used in the form of magnesium orotate, 100 to 200 mg per day. The patient should also aim to eat magnesium-rich food: bananas, cashew nuts, soya products, wheat bran, oatflakes, etc.

Therapeutic enemas

At the beginning enemas are given daily, increasing in volume; in our centre colonic irrigation is also carried out as an alternative. On the first day the enema consists of approximately 300 ml of weak, lukewarm camomile tea, usually with approximately 1⁄2 a measuring spoonful of Alkala N. After this the volume of the enema is gradually increased each day up to maximum of one litre, at which point two enemas are administered each day. According to the localisation of the main pain, the enema must be instilled higher, then slower, or less high and instead several times. 20 to 30 drops of Notakehl 5X are generally added at each instillation. The instillation is carried out with the simple 'Klysopumpe' and a size 18 single-use catheter for men.

Camomile tea is given as an enema only for one or two days because it dries out the mucous membrane and is low in acid. Afterwards the enemas which are given are of a special tea mixture made up to Dr. Karsch's recipe: this is a mixture of crushed fennel (2 parts), juniper (2 parts), aloe powder (1 part) and foenum gracum (fenugreek - 1 part). This mixture is left to stand for about 10 minutes over gentle heat. After it has cooled Notakehl 5X drops and Alkala N are added to the extract. Enemas using this liquid have a particularly stimulating effect on the liver and detoxicating effect. In some enema prescriptions approximately 20 ml of linseed oil is added at the end of the final enema.

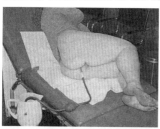

Fig 1
A patient is given a
theraputic enema

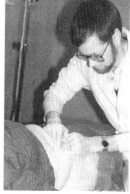

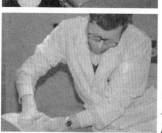

Fig 2 & 3
A doctor gives a special massage to a
patient with intestinal disease

Therapeutic acid-alkaline balance

In the majority of chronic inflammatory diseases there is over-acidification of the tissues which gives rise to an increase in the acid secretion of the mucous membranes. These in turn irritate the surface of the mucous membrane, which is why we buffer the enteral excretion of acid with the help of the enemas and so restrict the re-absorption of the acid. At the same time Alkala N is mostly given orally as a effective alkaline. The problems of disorders in the acid-base metabolism cannot be dealt with more fully here. I recommend the book "Praxis des Säure-Basen-Haushalts" (The practice of the acid-base metabolism) by Worlitschek which is full of insights.

Treatment with medication

The building up of symbiosis by means of medication is carried out on two fronts. It is begun with Notakehl, 1 tablet twice daily. In addition Notakehl can also be prescribed with 5 to 10 drops in the enema liquid. After 3 or 4 days we combine this with Fortakehl, 1 tablet twice daily. Only after the acute symptoms have subsided do we turn to Albicansan, 1 capsule daily, and/or Pefrakehl, 1 capsule daily – over a period of about another 10 days.

Only after this do we proceed to long-term treatment with Sankombi, 10 drops twice daily, or alternatively Mucokehl and Nigersan tablets, preferable in adults. Here the Mucokehl tablets are best given in the mornings as a yin medication and the Nigersan tablets are best taken in the late evening or at night as a yang medication.

In a series of stool investigations Dr. Werthmann has been able to show that the course of therapy described above leads to an increase in the number of physiological intestinal flora and to a reduction in the candida population, and in its effect can be compared with control of the symbiosis. In individual cases this can also be supported at the start by a 2 – or 3-week course of treatment with Symbioflor 1, 20 drops twice daily or Bioflorin, 1 tablet twice daily.

In cases of chronic colitis (Ulcerative Colitis or Crohn's disease) we mostly give an additional course of enzyme therapy, e.g. with Wobenzym, 1/2 tsp. 3 times daily, or with Kombucha tea. If at the start there are strong indications of inflammation, we prescribe Traumeel additionally in the form of tablets, injections, or added to the enema. In individual cases and as an addition, neural therapy (segment therapy) has also proved its worth, with administration of Notakehl and/or Traumeel.

As for the necessary immunological therapy, we start from the assumption that with colitis, and also with chronic recurrent diverticulitis, there is an accompanying disorder of the intestinal mucous membrane which again puts a strain on the intestinal defences. This shows up as a disorder of the intestinal lymph node system, including the important Peyer's patches. This makes the disturbance field of the intestinal mucous membrane into a focus, putting strain on the whole organism and with consequent weakening of the immune system and an increase in the general tendency towards disease and recurrent infections, etc. Intestinal allergies are also becoming more common as the cause of chronic inflammatory diseases. This is shown in work by Professor A. Rost and from our own observations using contact regulation thermography.

For these reasons we always combine the treatment of colitis and recurrent diverticulitis with an immunological stimulation therapy with Sanum remedies. At the beginning Rebas 4X is injected i.m. daily, but possibly also combined with neural therapy and the use of Notakehl, as already explained. This treatment continues for 1 or 2 weeks. Then follows improvement of peroral stimulation using Recarcin and Utilin in capsule form, with one capsule of each being given per week in the early morning on different, preferably non-consecutive days (e.g. on Sundays and Wednesdays). From the third to fourth week onwards, the triple combination of Utilin, Recarcin and Latensin is given, 1 capsule of each per week.

If there are allergic factors, e.g. a food allergy, atopy, an allergic lymphatic diathesis in iris diagnosis or problems with the joints, each month from about the fourth week we give one i.m. injection of Utilin "S" weak or one capsule of Utilin "S" strong orally: Utilin, Recarcin and Latensin are then not given that week.

With the complex therapy described here we have been able to treat successfully all the named cases of diverticulitis and also individual cases of serious colitis (Crohn's disease) in our outpatients' clinic. There were recurrences, mostly connected with a faulty diet and generally in situations where there was an excess of acid. In one case, it was possible to determine by means of colonoscopy that a previously impassable inflammatory sigma stenosis had disappeared. Antibiotics were only prescribed once and for a very short period; because of the need to travel during an acute recurrence of the condition, 100 mg of Doxycyclin was given as an exception.

Dr. Thomas Rau, m.d.
Paracelsus Klinik Lustmühle,
9062 Lustmühle (bei St.Gallen)
Switzerland

Lecture given at the 1993 Sanum Therapy Conference
Published in Sanum Post No. 23 1993

"BASIC" THERAPY FOR
INFLAMMATORY RHEUMATIC DISEASES

1. De-Acidification >> = Obligatory!

>> • Diet animal proteins, basic soup, sugar
>> • Minerals: magnesium/calcium 2 x 250-500 mg
>> • **Base supply** *Alkala N*
   • Lactic acid
   • (folic acid 15-30 mg/ day)

2. Alteration /Immune System "Stimulation"
   • Intestinal Cleansing
   • Citric acid
   • Quinone (Heel)
>> • Peyer's Patches extract 4X 3 x 1 -> 2 x 1 for months!
>> • Utilin strong, 1 capsule/week
   • *Bacillus firmus* strong, 1 capsule/week
   • *Bacillus cereus* strong, 1 capsule/week
   • Cupping, segmental neural therapy, etc
>> • *Fasting, Werthmann Diet*

3. Milieu Therapy
   • Begin with : *Penicillium chrysogenum* 5X 2-5 tablets once a day
>> • Then *Mucor racemosus* or *Mucor racemosus /
   Aspergillus niger* for one year!

4. Substitution
A Antioxidants -> INHIBIT INFLAMMATION

>> Vitamin E	500-1500 IU/day	
Vitamin C	1-3g/day	
DL-methionine		
Selenium	50-200µg	
Zinc	20-50mg 3 tid	
Manganese		

>> EVENING PRIMROSE OIL   2-4 grams/day
B Pain Therapy
Vitamin B6   100-300mg/day
Magnesium orotate   250-500 mg 3 tid
Wobenzyme
Vitamin E
DL-methionine
>> Alcohol, Nicotine   Forbidden!
Histamine stop
(DL-phenylalanine   750 mg 3 tid)

Table 12

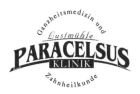

19

Osteoporosis – a misunderstood ‚popular' illness

Osteoporosis (brittle bones) is erroneously commonly equated with calcium deficiency and people try to treat it accordingly. However the results of classic medical school treatment are extremely poor, since they start from this assumption of a calcium deficiency. Osteoporosis actually involves a reduction in the bone trabeculae, in other words impaired structural metabolism in the organic and anorganic bone mass.

Bones are built up of trabeculae, which comprise strands of connective tissue, with enclosed bone cells. Around these strands of connective tissue and between the cells, calcium substances (calcium phosphate and calcium hydroxyapatite) are stored. The bone-producing cells (osteoblasts) and the bone-resorbing cells (osteoclasts) counterbalance each other.

In young bodies the structural forces predominate, the metabolism of the child is basally adjusted, the circulation in the bones is very active. In the child and the young person the bone is elastic and this is due to the richness of the connective tissue and elastic fibres in the bone. The proportion of anorganic calcium in the elastic, healthy bone in relation to the organic, connective-tissue, cellular substance is small. Thus the bone is hard and resistant to compression, but also slightly elastic. With increasing age the bone becomes more brittle and this is due to the fact that the connective tissue parts, which need to be constantly renewed, are produced less copiously, the proportion of bone trabeculae is reduced and the relative proportion of calcium tends to increase. The bone becomes weaker, but above all more brittle.

In **bone densitometry** tests commonly carried out today (measurement of bone density), the bone appears to be weakened and to have lowered calcium, since these tests only measure the density but not the number of trabeculae, which actually ensure the bone function. Thus people are erroneously of the opinion that the reduced level of calcium is the cause of the problem of increased brittleness of the bones in old age.

On the subject of bone scans it should also be mentioned that in tall, leptosomatic female patients, bone densitometry is not meaningful, since these patients have a constitutionally slimmer build, with longitudinal trabeculae predominating over the transverse trabeculae and therefore fall below the average bone density of subjects of the same weight even when their bone stability is intact. It is precisely these often willowy patients who frequently have the diagnosis of osteoporosis thrust upon them.

Thus the standard values for female patients of the same age are not the ideal densitometric values for leptosomatic patients and not those of cachexic patients either.

If one studies the tissue histologically however, one can see that in older subjects, as a result of a massive metabolic shift, the bone contains fewer trabeculae, which individually are normally to even excessively calcified but have become brittle and fragile.

Therapy for age-related osteoporosis therefore needs to start from bone metabolism and production, in other words the organic part of the bone, and not from the calcium content.

Female hormones and osteoporosis:

It is well known that women are more inclined to osteoporosis than men. This has been attributed to the reduction in oestrogen after the menopause. But this is not correct, it is the reduction in all the female hormones, in particular progesterone, which is the cause of the increased bone loss in women of menopausal age.

It has been shown that increased bone loss among women of about 1-2% of the bone mass per year actually begins 5-10 years before the menopause, in other words at a time when the periods often first start to become somewhat more irregular (see diagram). However at that time oestrogen hormone production is still completely normal and it is only

The
Dr. Rau's Diet For
Whole Body Healing

SWISS

SECRET

to Optimal Health

Build a
better body
cell by cell

Thomas Rau, M.D.
with Susan Wyler

Turn your life around with whole body healing.

THE SWISS SECRET
to Optimal Health

For the first time, world-renowned physician
Dr. Thomas Rau explains the secret of Swiss biological
medicine—natural healing based on the latest research
and proven principles of well-being. This program
will allow you to:

- Purify your body
- Strengthen your immune system
- Encourage healing
- Prevent illness
- Feel young and energetic—in body and mind

With an effective nutrition program, complete menu
plans, and more than 100 delicious recipes, you can
begin to turn your health and your life around—now.

Available Now

978-0-425-21393-3/$23.95

penguin.com

progesterone production which is decreasing. It is at the time of progesterone reduction that osteoporosis begins. <u>By administering oestrogens therefore one can at most halt the osteoporosis but not reverse it. A reversal of osteoporosis can only be achieved by supplying natural progesterone</u>, or even better the precursors of natural progesterone, from which the body itself manufactures its hormones. A cream made from the South American wild yam, containing diosgenin, produces astonishing success in this situation. Diosgenin is a precursor of human hormone synthesis, contained in various plants, which allows the body to produce its own hormone (Pro-Gest cream, Info from Author).

The main cause of osteoporosis is on the one hand a reduced bone metabolism, due to circulatory disorders and ageing, but on the other hand excessive acidification and protein, which to a large extent are nutrition-related. Excessive acidification is caused by poor nutrition, among other things the consumption of protein-rich foods, above all animal proteins. It has been shown that races with vegetarian diets (Japan and inland China and Africa) display no osteoporosis or almost none. Similarly women of these races have scarcely any menopausal hot flushes, which are also an expression of hormone misuse and excess acidification).

Our diet, which is customarily too rich in protein, leads to a concentration of amino acids, which we cannot utilise and which act as acids. (The average Swiss eats about 120g of protein daily, but can only metabolise and absorb 40-60g, so that there is a gigantic surplus). The body tries to bind these surplus amino acids and surplus proteins by neutralising them with calcium and storing them somewhere in the body, e.g. as hardenings of the connective tissue, deposits in the tissues or arteriosclerosis. The calcium needed for this is drawn from the bones (see diagram 2) and this leads to a loss of calcium from the bones. However at the same time magnesium and other trace elements are taken from the cartilage and bone, which can lead to heart and arthrosis problems. (Diagram: later consequences of excess acidification)

Risk factors for brittle bones:

– **Constitution**: There are people, particularly women, who have inherited a predisposition to decalcification of the bones or carry it with them in their constitution. These are predominantly slim, sinewy, prematurely greying women, usually with a dry skin, sensitive to cold, inclined to headaches and back pain, tension. These people, who often benefit from exercise, sport, heat applications and energy input, need to pay increased attention to stress and keep themselves warm, eat mainly hot meals and practise sport.

– **Hormones**: Women who never have children run an increased risk of osteoporosis. Women who took the contraceptive pill over a long period during their child-bearing years have higher risk of osteoporosis, since their own oestrogen synthesis and progesterone synthesis are somewhat reduced and the supply of oestrogens also makes the cellular utilization of thyroid hormones more difficult.

– **Smoking**: Smoking over-acidifies and increases the risk of osteoporosis quite massively. With a nicotine habit bone circulation is massively reduced and this affects the bone metabolism.

– **Sport/Exercise**: The less the exercise, the higher the risk of osteoporosis. Daily exercise, the „heating from within and circulatory stimulation", is therefore extremely important.

– **Nutrition**: The poorer the plant nutrition, above all from fresh raw plant products, the higher the risk of osteoporosis and the higher the quantity of animal proteins (see above) the higher the risk of developing osteoporosis. Dr.Rau has therefore developed a diet which is very appropriate for osteoporosis, since it is basically very rich in minerals and nourishes the intestinal flora (see below).

– **Condition of the intestinal flora and mineral absorption**:
In his intestine man has more bacteria cells than in his entire body. These bacteria perform a very intensive metabolism and prepare the nutrients in a form in which they can be absorbed, by organic binding.

But they also bind toxins and heavy metals, which could have a blocking effect on cell renewal in the body. Recent research has increasingly shown that the intactness of the intestinal flora is of the utmost significance for calcium uptake. On the one hand the intestinal flora produces vitamin K, which supports these organic binding processes. Only with good intact intestinal flora can calcium be sufficiently absorbed, which is why an important part of osteoporosis therapy involves building up the intestinal flora.

Therapy for Osteoporosis therefore comprises:

1. Deacidification: low-protein nutrition. Meat or fish at most twice a week. As few dairy products as possible, since these have an excessively high protein content. In particular avoid yoghurt, ,quark' and cheese. Use milk at most as an additive in coffee, which should also preferably be cut down. The calcium present in high quantities in milk is only poorly absorbed. Eat lots of vegetables.
   To deacidify the body: take the base powder continuously: either Alkala N (from ebi-pharm) or – somewhat less effective – some other base powder.

2. **Reduction of risk factors**: give up nicotine, take up daily exercise, sport, walking, hiking, cycling. Stimulating the metabolism by boosting the circulation is extremely important.
   Wine-drinking: alcoholic drinks over-acidify the body. Wine taken in quantities of more than one glass a day puts a strain on the liver owing to its alcohol content. The liver metabolises oestrogens and has an indirect influence on bone metabolism. People who drink alcohol regularly are more inclined to osteoporosis.

3. **Stimulating the metabolism**: the main thrust of the therapy (apart from the strict deacidification and diet) of the Paracelsus Klinik lies in stimulating bone metabolism with bleeding, massage, above all along the vertebral column, administering medicines which boost the metabolism and circulation in the bones: with neural therapy and subcutaneous injections calcium fluoratum, silica products, Latensin and viscum (mistletoe) remedies are injected along the spine. All of

these help to build up the bone trabeculae and thus lead to a strengthening of the bones and increased elasticity. The pains associated with osteoporosis, which are usually severe, mostly disappear completely within a few weeks of this therapy.

Natural progesterone / <u>natural hormone</u>: There are creams made from yam roots and other phyto-oestrogen-containing plants, from which the body can make its own gestagens (progesterone). After using them for several weeks the hormone metabolism usually normalises and bone incorproration can be enhanced (Pro Gest cream). Natural precursors of oestrogens and gestagens are contained in many plants (see the attached list). This therapy not only leads to an improvement in the bone structure, it also eliminates, in most cases, the extremely irksome hot flushes experienced by menopausal women, which have similar origins.

Very recently we have acquired, at the Paracelsus Klinik, **<u>natural hormones in capsule form for oral administration</u>**. They are also made from so-called „phyto-oestrogens" and have exactly the same organic chemical formula as the body's own hormones and therefore do NOT lead to a suppression of the natural hormone function. They stimulate the bone-building osteoblasts (bone-forming cells). These phyto-hormones have been very popular in the USA for years and have proved their worth superbly. Their greatest advantage is that they do NOT increase womens risk of cancer, but rather reduce it, since they contain the cancer-inhibiting estriol and progesterone. Their effect on bone formation is striking.

Calcium:

Theoretically humans need about ½ to 1 gramme of calcium a day. However it is not usually the supply which is the problem, since that is easily achieved, the limiting factor is calcium synthesis and absorption. The calcium supply is most beneficial when it is obtained from organic structures: calcium from shellfish, e.g. Weleda bone-building calcium. This can be far better incorporated into the bones than inorganic calcium. However to improve bone structure it is above all silica, e.g.obtained from horsetail (equisetum) which should be administered, it is the organic structural agent in mineral therapy and homeopathy.

Calcium resorption is improved with vitamin D, we recommend ViDe drops, 3-10 drops per day.

Intestinal flora and calcium uptake:

In osteoporosis therapy it is not a question of the calcium supply, but of mineral uptake in the body and calcium absorption into the organic bone structure. This „organic" uptake is decisively affected also by the intestinal flora. It is therefore of the greatest importance to build up the intestinal flora:

- The intestinal flora is nourished by cellulose-rich food: raw food, finely grated
- The intestinal flora is strengthened by vitamin K (Kanavit, 3-10mg/day)
- Intestinal flora-boosting products (isopathics such as Sankombi, Fortakehl etc., but also the actual bacterial remedies: Bioflorin or Vitabiosa)

A tremendous improvement in osteoporosis was observed in the USA when the therapy involved the administration of vitamin K, which had prevoiusly only been known for blood coagulation problems. In studies 10mg Kanavit (10 drops) per day for 1 year improved the average bone density by 3%.

Biological medicines for the treatment of osteoporosis:

Hormone replacement: before the doctor even considers prescribing hormones the female hormones AND the hormone precursors cholesterin and DHEA should be measured – preferably in the first week and the last week of the cycle, but absolutely in the days BEFORE the expected period – but also the pituitary hormones FSH and LH which stimulate the ovaries. Then one can see which hormones are required or where the „knot" is: in fact it is usually progesterone and not oestrogens, though the doctors are so quick to reach for the latter. However one can also see whether the body wants to stimulate hormones itself. In these cases women respond particularly well to the natural precursors. However, frequently the cause is a weakness in the pituitary gland, where it is not stimulating the ovaries at all. In these cases the low hormone levels are due to toxic disorders, most often heavy metals or other cytotoxins, or to the liver. (A heavy metal load on the pituitary gland and the ovaries is also the commonest cause of sterility in women).

In any case: the problems of alteration are not oestrogen problems but usually progesterone problems or underlying deficiencies and enzyme blocks! Administration of oestrogen in isolation, as it is unfortunately most often administered, is detrimental and usually misguided.

There are many hormone products, most of which are oestrogen-laden and a few (older) are actually pure oestrogen (e.g. Premarin). Apart from the biological versions obtained from plants, they are derived from the urine of pregnant horses, which is very rich in hormones. These hormones are then somewhat chemically altered (so that they can be patented by the companies and also produce a viable product). Admittedly they still have the hormonal effect but they cause a lot of side effects and are actually carcinogenic: e.g. the oestrogen estradiol (= Premarin among many others) of the gestagen Medroxyprogesterone acetate (as in depot Provera among others). These categories also include all contraceptive pills, which actually suppress the woman's own hormone production, in other words actually do precisely the wrong thing (at least these drugs are today usually low dosage). **Estron**, a form of oestrogen which is present in large quantities in horses, is normally not present in women or not more than 8% at most and is actually a strong trigger for breast cancer.

Other therapies to improve bone metabolism:

The natural hormones: in the USA they have hormones extracted from plants which match the human hormones exactly and are composed in proportions which match those of the woman. (e.g. Bi-oestrogen / or natural progesterone (ProGest). They do not provoke the side effects of hormone therapy, such as adiposity, venous problems, thread veins, mood swings, high blood pressure, loss of libido etc.

The hormone precursors produced by the body itself, such as glutathione, diosgenin, DHEA, pregnenolone, are even better, as they can specifically boost poor endogenous hormone production, even in elderly women. Since the steroidal hormones, as described above, have far wider effects than merely sexual, one can also influence other hormones favourably with them such as adrenalin, endogenous cortisone and serotonin (blood pressure and circulation), thus tackling e.g. arthritis, skin diseases, allergies etc. biologically!

Your doctor for biological medicine or your homeopathically-inclined gynaecologist can advise you.

All these hormone precursors, but also the right trace elements, vitamins and high class fatty acids, can be obtained in the **Paracelsus Klinik in Lustmühle**, which is the first institution of its kind in Switzerland to investigate natural hormones, import them from the USA and make them available to their patients.

The success of this natural hormone therapy is striking: even problems such as libido disorders, impotence disorders (in men) and even prostate cancer and breast cancer can be successfully treated with them, naturally in conjunction with other biological therapies.

In contrast to the synthetic hormones, which are often carcinogenic, the natural hormones e.g. endogenous progesterone, are precisely cancer-inhibiting and promote the building of healthy tissue such as e.g. bone mass.

In the USA this form of natural hormones is well established in medicine and is actually routine. One can only attribute to the massive advertising and „information" fed to doctors here by the pharmaceutical industry the fact that these products are only known to, and administered by, a very few doctors.

A few **biological remedies for the menopause / osteoporosis** which are available in the Paracelsus Klinik in Lustmühle:

Natural hormones:

– DHEA 25mg capsules 60 units

– Bi-estrogen 2.5mg / progesterone 100mg capsules 60 units (cash payment)
(Estriol 2.5% / Estradiol 2.5mg / Progesterone 100mg per capsule)

- Estriol 0.05%, vaginal ointment 50g tube with applicator (cash payment)

- Pregnenolone 10mg capsules 60 (gelatine-free)

- Pregnenolone 30mg capsules 60 (gelatine-free)

- Progesterone 50mg capsules 60

- Progesterone 100mg capsules 60

- Pro-Gest Body Cream 60ml tube

- Testosterone 10mg capsules 60

- Androstenadion spray 2.5mg/shot 60ml

Medicines for osteroporosis:

For prophylaxis or even treatment of manifest osteoporosis there are many natural products available. One should distinguish between homeopathic and orthomolecular remedies. The former generally boost bone and tooth regeneration in the body on the energy-information level (they are all „substance-free"). The latter provide the body with the minerals and vitamins necessary to build up and maintain the bones. In degenerative bone disease long term treatment lasting years and consistent dairy-free or low-milk diets are very important!

Complex homeopathic remedies:

Oss Regen from Pekana: homeopathic-spagyric complex remedy from the plant and mineral realm. To be used where bone density is reduced, for periostitis, slipped discs etc. (Oss Regen is freely available in drop form, 50 or 100ml).

Osteoheel from Heel: homeopathic remedy from the plant, mineral and animal realm. This remedy is suitable for alleviating periostitis and other bone diseases. (Osteoheel requires a prescription and is supplied in tablet form).

Restorative calcium 1 and 2 from Weleda: dynamic anthroposophical remedy. Weleda restorative calcium comprises mineral, animal and vegetable components. This remedy is the only one on the market to consist of two different powders to be taken morning and evening, totally adapted to the body's requirements and circadian rhythm! (This combination pack is available as 2x50g, 2x100g or a 500g pack).

Urticalcin from Bioforce: homeopathic remedy from the plant and mineral kingdom. Indicated for calcium deficiency manifestations to boost bone structure, brittle finger nails etc.
(Urticalcin is available in tablet form).

Equisetum ceres: this horsetail or equisetum remedy is perfectly suited to guide and promote the structural forces in the body. It not only influences the building up of the bones but also helps to cleanse the connective tissue and promote kidney activity – it is precisely these additional properties which make Equisetum Ceres the ideal concomitant medication in any osteoporosis treatment (available as drops).

Trace elements and vitamins which boost the regenerative forces:

Dolomite from Burgerstein: Dolomite chewable tablets contain, in physiological terms, the ideal combination of two parts of calcium to 1 part magnesium. Thus it is perfectly suited to supplying the body with these minerals which it needs for building up and maintaining the bones. (Available as chewable tablets).

At present (unfortunately) there is no registered product available on the market which contains vitamin D3, vitamin K, phosphorus, vitamin C, vitamin E, silicic acid, zinc and selenium in addition to calcium and magnesium, which would provide the ideal combination and availability. Such a combination would be desirable for preventing and relieving bone diseases.

However we at Paracelsus Klinik can already offer you these important vitamins and minerals in homeopathic and orthomolecular quality and we also have the corresponding natural hormones available for you.

Dr. Thomas Rau, M.D.
Paracelsus Klinik Lustmühle,
9062 Lustmühle (bei St.Gallen)
Switzerland

Daniel Ackermann,
Chartered graduate pharmacist ETH

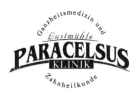

20

Calcium – from Childhood to Old Age

In recent years, Calcium has come very much to the attention of the layman, mainly through advertisements and background information from dairy organizations but also "patient groups" for osteoporosis, behind which stands the pharmaceutical industry (hormones and osteoporosis medicines), to a large extent, as backers.

Calcium (with the chemical indication Ca = calcium) is a mineral substance which occurs in large quantities in the earth and is important and essential for many bodily functions but is only available to us from external sources.

Calcium is also the mineral found in the largest quantities in the body. It is esp. found in the bones, partly inorganically and partly in organically-bound form: calcium phosphate, calcium apatite, calcium carbonate.

It partly determines the hardness of the bones, but only in connection with the organic and flexible fibers of connecting tissues. Calcium alone would be too hard, too likely to split, like gypsum, and only strengthens as a component of the total organic structure of the bone.

Two illnesses, in which calcium is not stored in the bones, are rachitis in children and osteomalacia in adults, both, fortunately, very rare diseases today. The bones have too large a portion of organic structures, are too flexible and not hard enough, however do not break. This, then, is a true problem of calcium intake and assimilation.

This is different with osteoporosis in aging humans, esp. aging woman. This is caused hormonally and constitutionally and is today, unfortunately, a very frequent illness.

With osteoporosis, **calcium is not the true problem,** but rather the decreased generation of organic bone structure, i.e., the connecting tissue part of the bone. The bone fibers, in this case, are decreased but too strongly calcified, which is why they become too brittle and often fracture. Under histological investigation, these bones appear "empty", with little bone structure. It is therefore necessary to redevelop these organic structures, by promoting the forces of regeneration. With women, this is usually accomplished by prescribing silicon (which promotes the regeneration of fibrous organic structure: common horse tail (Equisetum arvense)), as well as by low-molecular, vegetable proteins, alkaline nutrition, and eventually – but only after testing the hormones with a biologically trained physician – by prescribing natural (not synthetic!!) progesterone, which stimulates the bone-developing osteoblasts.

Under certain conditions, calcium is depleted from the bones. This is then usually the true cause of osteoporosis and not the lack of calcium!

The main cause is an over-acidification of the organism, i.e. the presence of too many acidic elements, esp. in the form of free, not assimilateable amino acids, as the result of a too protein-rich nutrition, but also the presence of too many organic acids, like phosphates, gluconate, lactate, ect.. These are present in large quantities in conserved foods, even in milk products, which are unreasonably recommended for the treatment of bone decalcification!

Calcium is a very valuable generator of alkalic elements, as it goes to and replaces the $H+$ ion (that is, the acid ion).

However, if too much calcium is used in the body for this acid-compensation, this leads to the calcifying of tissue, so-called arterial sclerosis (calcifying of arterial walls), the tendons and connective tissue (soft tissue rheumatism) and intervertebral disks (back problems, herniated discs, etc.).

It is thus wrong, to think that one can counter the aging processes by intake of calcium. One meets this with correct nutrition and exercise (see below).

Calcium still has, however, some very important other functions: As a catalyst for many metabolic processes and as an exchange ion for cell activity. The vitality of the cells, i.e. the electrical potential of the cell membranes, is developed through an exchange of magnesium and calcium in the cell walls. In addition, calcium and magnesium adjust the hearts activity, as well as all unconscious, vegetative functions, in co-operation with potassium and sodium, which must likewise also be in equilibrium.

Calcium is also necessary for blood clotting.

The calcium exchange within the body follows a very complicated hormonal automatic control-loop of parathyroid hormone (formed in the parathyroid glands) and calcitonin.

Today, "civilized" people are usually over-acidic, and often have a lack of magnesium, which is only more heavily aggravated by unreasonable consumption of calcium. In addition, they often have too much sodium (from salt and meat) and a lack of potassium.

Only vegetable foods (if possible, 1–2/3 raw) replace all these necessary minerals in the correct proportions.

Milk and milk products are very rich in calcium, however, this calcium is useless, since an excess of phosphorus and esp. a strong excess of milk protein, binds the calcium and therefore makes it inaccessible for the cells and bones.

Milk and milk products are therefore not suitable for and are to be advised against, in the treatment of osteoporosis and it's cause, over-acidity. In Chinese Medicine, milk is considered to have a detrimental effect on lymph and to be acidifying! We know that today, over half (certain studies claim 2/3) of western people react allergically, in one form or another, to milk proteins. Also, we must consider that a milk cow today gives approx. 3x as much milk as the best cows 40 years ago. This kind of milk is however, no longer as rich in content by far as in former times. Another problem is that these poor cows are nourished, in a way quite alien to their species, with "power foods", which frequently contain meal from the corpses of dead animals, thus promoting infections. And besides: why don't the poor cows get bone weaknesses, when they give daily 20–40 liters of milk? Because they eat alkaline, i.e. nourish them-selves with green vegetables!!

Particularly children should not receive milk products, as they are over-acidifying, work allergy-promoting and very frequently cause immune disturbances and a tendency to infections. Don't let yourselves be dazzled by the advertisements of the milk and "functional" food industry, which even adds, unreasonably, inorganic calcium to the milk.

Children may take rice milk or soya milk as a substitute. However, we do not recommend milk-type beverages anyway, but rather tea or simply water. Under no circumstances drink artificially sweet beverages, such as Coca Cola, Fanta, Zitro, etc., since they can contain phosphates and make children nervous and over-acid. The so-called "light beverages", whose sugar is replaced by Aspartame (an artificial sweetener), is still worse!

One can receive Calcium in quite sufficient measures, if the body is neutralized (take initially the alkaline powder Alkala N from Sanum) by vegetables, which contain the other mineral substances evenly, which are missing in the correct measure in the milk:

- carrots, beans, flax seed, soja foods, whole-meal bread, spinach, broccoli, salads, sauerkraut
- almonds, hazel nuts, cashew nuts, macadamia nuts, dried fruits
- eggs
- with cheese, we recommend non-allergenic sheep's milk cheese, which is richer in minerals and calcium: front-runner: Pecorino, so 1–2 x per week 50–100g

It is important to know that all phosphate-rich, acidic foods reduce calcium absorption: sausages, sugar foods, sweet beverages, ketchup, melting cheese, chocolate, all processed products.

Further data in the list "Calcium maintenance".

Let us again mention, that it is not the calcium content but the proportions of mineral substances and alkalinity that is important! Calcium assimilation – similar to iron – is the problem and not the calcium supply (nobody would think to eat iron splinters with an iron deficiency, since these could not be assimilated)!!

The assimilation of calcium into the body depends on vitamin D and, in the intestines, the intestinal bacteria. When the intestinal bacteria is intact – again, also promoted by vegetable raw foods – the calcium absorption into the blood is much better. Oil rich meals, like olive oil, cashew nuts, sea-fish, as well as wheat germ oil, flax seed oil, contain very much vitamin D and, among other things, unsaturated fatty acids which should always be taken in quite large quantities, since they are important for children and their cranial nerve-cell generation.

So, one sees that the "calcium problem" can not be solved only mechanistically through the addition of calciu m! And again: no milk – especially with children – and do not even think of Yoghurt at all!

CALCIUM

How much calcium does a person need daily?
adults:	800 mg
women in menopause:	1'000 mg – 1'200 mg
women after menopause:	1'500 mg

food, that contains calcium: *(mg per 100 g)*

alga (brown)	1000	sunflower seeds	100
sesame	783	wholegrain bread	95
cabbage dried	375	onion	160
linseeds	260	beans	150
carrots	255	spinach	85
almonds	250	apricots dried	80
hazelnuts	225	lentil	75
green beans dried	195	walnuts	70
soyflour	195	wheat seeds, sprouts	70
fig dried	190	broccoli	65
parsley	145	rolled oats	65
chives	130	tomatoes	60
cacao	115	crisp bread	55
green cabbage	110	horseradish	50
white beans	105	sauerkraut	50
fennel	100	celery	50

Dr. Thomas Rau, M.D.
Paracelsus Klinik Lustmühle,
9062 Lustmühle (bei St.Gallen)
Switzerland

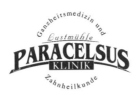

21

Menopause and Female Hormones: the Biological Medicine Approach

Holistic or better termed "biological" medicine, approaches diseases, not only by suppressing their symptoms but by eliminating their causes. It's goal is to bring the body back into the condition of self regulation, in order to be able to overcome it's weaknesses with it's own resources.

Are you a woman around 50 and coming into menopause? Then someone has surely already recommended that you to take female hormones. These would protect you from osteoporosis and also calm your nerves. Not only that but also your skin remains more beautiful and, much more besides! Easy said, easy done? Already taken estrogen? But what are the long-term effects?

Some background information or "what your doctor didn't tell you":
The whole problem (i.e. natural complaints) around female but also male, age-related changes, is an expression of changing hormone production and can be solved far better, if not completely, with biological methods:

THE YEARS BEFORE BLEEDING STOPS

The normal rhythm of hormone production and the quantity of the prog-esterone, decreases approx. 5–8 years before the periods stop. Progesterone is a growth hormone, which not only makes a pregnancy possible, but works also as a general growth hormone, strengthening the whole body, a "rejuvenating hormone" as it were. It corresponds to testosterone in men, which is responsible for potency and erectile function, in addition to general endurance, strength and muscle power.

From the time of the decrease of progesterone levels, the process of bone formation also decreases slowly, which can lead to back and bone problems. In addition, in this phase, the cholesterine levels will frequently be increased! Why? Because it is the initial or intermediate stage of the progesterone synthesis and the cholesterine processing enzymes or the trace elements necessary for it, are missing. During this time, women can very much be helped if they are given the components which improve progesterone production:

Polyunsaturated fatty acids such as are contained in vegetable oils: linseed oil, evening primrose oil, cold-pressed olive oil, wheat-germ oil. There are also special oil mixtures (in the USA the have characteristically funny names like "women's help", with us in Switzerland "perfect balance oil"). Another possibility is **vitamin-e and magnesium** and selenium, as well as (esp. for men) zinc, which promotes the hormone-forming enzymes. All these substances have other good effects.

We are thereby also helped on other levels, from which we would otherwise not profit with the usual hormone pills, which would indeed be harmful to us!

Selenium

- is the best documented cancer prophylactic for women.
  Unsaturated fatty acids also make the skin supple, help against concentration disturbances and depression. **Zinc** helps the prostate with men and detoxes (also like selenium) from heavy metals, which are so often a secondary problem! **Vitamin E** in a dosage over 400 – 800 I.E.

- is both a stimulator of the body's own hormone-producing enzymes, in addition to **anti-oxidants** which helps with the neutralization of cell-own and carcinogenic-free radicals.

Some vegetable materials are well suitable for the support of hormone synthesis and also against the symptoms of menopause: They are contained in some of the following, proven plant preparations:

Alchemilla comp. (Ceres): One of the best products available. Those who know Ceres products, know they meet the highest requirements which are placed on their raw materials, manual processing, special extraction, storage etc.. This makes possible the enormously low dosage of daily only 3 times 5 drops. Alchemilla comp. drops work with psychosomatic complaints, in menopause, with hot flushes, with dysmenorrhea and also with pre-menstrual syndrome. (available as drops, 20ml).

KLIFEM (Pekana): is a compound from 8 components from the plant, animal and mineral realm and spagyrically / homeopathically processed. Klifem is effective with such menopause complaints as hot flushes, psychological stress etc.. Klifem should be proportioned daily 3 times to 20 drops each. (available as drops in 50 and 100ml).

Viburnum comp. (Heel): Homeopathic Complex Remedy with 14 components from the plant, animal and mineral realm. The components are finely coordinated with the function of the mucous membranes, the female sex organs, cramp-like complaints of hollow organs, physical and psychological unrest and nervousness etc. Vibunum comp. drops are to be proportioned 3 time daily to 20 drops. (available as ampoules or drops to 30, 100 and 1000ml).

Menosan (Bioforce): Homeopathic Complex Remedy with 6 compo-nents from the plant and animal realm. Equally effective with menopause complaints, pain around the female abdomen organs, sleep disturbances etc.. Dosage also 3 times daily, 10 to 20 drops regularly. (available as drops or tablets).

Chasteberry (Vitex agnus castus) and **black cohosh** (Cimicifuga) repre-sent nowadays the most usual Phytopharmaca for the treatment of female complaints. Both single and combination preparations of both plants exist (primarily for the treatment of Premenstrual Syndrome).

With chasteberry, there are two products available in Switzerland: **Agnolyt** from Madaus as tablets or drops or **Emoton** from Tentan AG. Chasteberry is offered as a single product in Switzerland under the following names: Cimifemin, Drosana Femicin, Remifemin, Alpinamed PMS drops. In combination with other plant based substances, a good dozen further products are available.

Well proved besides: **Klimaktoplant** tablets, **Mulimen** drops or homeopathic/anthroposophic organ extracts, such as **Ovarium comp.** from Heel or Wala etc..

NUTRITION is very important.

Vegetables, soja, potatoes, peas and fish promote hormone synthesis, whereas meat, milk and sugar suppress this and promote lymph congestion and swelling, which are so often a problem anyway. Fruits, but only eaten in the morning, drain the body of excess water. Particularly good are: apricots, apples and pears (peeled). Nuts contain lots of magnesium and calcium. Balanced acid-neutralizing mineral formulations (Alen/Alkala, etc..) make the body more alkaline. Progesterone is only formed in an alkaline environment.

SOME REMARKS ON OSTEOPOROSIS AND SYMPTOMS OF MENOPAUSE:

Women between 40 and 50 years old are very frequently fooled into believing that they should start to take hormones because of the threat of osteoporosis, particularly if they belong to one of the so-called risk groups: smokers, childless women, slim types or if osteoporosis has already occurred in the family.

"Estrogen would help to strengthen the bones again". This is unfortunately not correct, since estrogen only slightly slows down bone degeneration and this has only been proven over a period of 2–3 years. Those elements that really support regenerative processes are progesterone and other elements like anti-acidic therapies, mineral salts, esp. silicon, zinc, manganese, and in certain cases also calcium.

The quantity of the body's own progesterone falls off in women approx. 5–8 years before menopause (absence of the period bleedings) and this often causes irregular bleedings and proportionally more estrogen. These high estrogen levels and age-based fluctuations account for the typical symptoms of menopause, like hot flushes, depressions, swellings and esp. weight gains, growth of myomas and the strong monthly bleedings!

Estrogens follow the acid principle and unfold their side-effects far stronger in the over-acidified body. Alkalines and alkaline nutrition make all these symptoms better, because progesterone follows the alkaline-developing principle.

Back to osteoporosis: It is progesterone which promotes bone-generation cells (osteoblasts). Also, bone-density reduction in women already takes place at a time in which the estrogen levels are still high.

The therapy of menopause symptoms and esp. the beginning of bone-density reduction is therefore: support of progesterone levels (i.e. Diosgenin or natural progesterone), anti-acid therapy and mineral-salt therapies (however not from milk, from which the calcium is not reabsorbed at all and which does not contain the other important minerals)

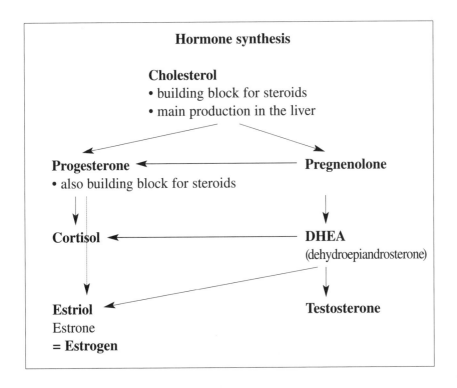

HORMONE REPLACEMENT

Before the physician thinks at all on a hormone treatment, he should – at best in the first week and in the last week of the cycle, certainly in the days before the expected period – measure the female hormones AND the hormone preliminary stages, cholesterol and DHEA, in addition to the ovary-stimulating hormones FSH and LH of the pituitary gland. Then, one sees which hormones are needed at all, or where the problem is: usually it is progesterone and not at all estrogen, which the physicians are so quick to administer. In addition, one sees whether the body would like to stimulate hormones. In these cases, women respond particularly well to the natural preliminary stages.

Frequently, however, it is a weakness of the pituitary gland that exists, which then does not stimulate the ovaries at all. In these cases, the low hormone levels are caused by toxic disturbances, usually heavy metals or other cellular poisons or the liver (heavy metal toxicity of the pituitary gland and the ovaries is also the most frequent cause for sterility in women).

Anyhow: the disturbances are not estrogen problems, but mostly progesterone problems or more deeply lying deficiencies and enzyme blockages! An isolated estrogen treatment, as unfortunately often happens, is harmful and usually wrong.

There are many **hormone preparations,** which are mostly estrogen and some (outdated) even pure estrogen preparations (e.g. Premarin). They are produced (except those of organic origin) from the urine of pregnant horses, which is very rich in hormones.

These hormones are then slightly changed chemically (so that the companies can patent them and make a profitable product). They still have the hormonal effect but have however, increased side effects and are even carcinogenic: e.g. the estrogen Estradiol (Premarin) or the gestagene medroxyprogesterone-acetate (Depot-Provera.) Also in this category are all contraceptive pills, which even suppress female hormone production, actually, exactly the wrong thing (today, at least, these preparations are usually dosed very low). Estrone, a form of estrogen, which is present to a considerable degree in horses, is normally not – or with maximally 8% – present in women and is even a strong promoter of breast cancer.

THE NATURAL HORMONES

In the USA, hormones are extracted from plants, which correspond exactly to human hormones and are mixed in proportions that especially fill women's needs (e.g. Bi-Estrogen or natural progesterone (Pro-Gest)). They have none of the side effects of the hormone therapy, for example: adiposity, varicose veins, spider veins, mood fluctuations, high blood pressure, loss of libido, etc.!

Still more ingenious are the hormonal preliminary stages of the body's own hormone production, like glutathione, diosgenin, DHEA, pregnanediol, which can support weak hormone production, even with older women.

Since the steroidal hormones, as described above, have far broader effects than only sexual ones, they can also favorably effect other hormones like adrenalin, cortisone-production and serotonin (blood pressure and blood circulation), and as such, treat arthritis, skin problems. allergies, etc. biologically!

Your physician for biological medicine or your naturopathically aligned gynecologist can advise you.

All these hormonal preliminary stages but also the correct trace-elements, vitamins and high-quality fatty-acids are all available in the Paracelsus Clinic, the first institution of this kind in Switzerland working with natural hormones, importing them from the USA and making them available for their female patients (Dr. Th. Rau, medical director and Dr. Harold Seiler, visiting gynecologist, of the Paracelsus Clinic Lustmühle).

This natural hormone therapy is proving a great success: even problems such as lack of libido, potency disturbances (with men), even prostate cancer and cancer of the breast can be treated successfully with it, naturally, when accompanied by other biological therapies. As apposed to synthetic hormones, which are often carcinogenic, natural hormones are, e.g. the body's own progesterone, almost cancer-restraining and promote the generation of healthy tissue and bone structure.

In the USA, this form of the natural hormone therapy is completely established in medicine and almost the routine. It is only because of massive advertising and the spreading of "information" to local physicians by the pharmaceutical industry, that these preparations are only known and used by very few physicians in Switzerland.

Some **biological preparations for menopause/osteoporosis,** which are available in the biological pharmacy of the Paracelsus Clinic Lustmühle:

Natural hormones:

- DHEA 25mg 60caps
- Biestrogen 2,5mg / progesterone 100mg 60caps (estriol 2,5mg / estradiol 2,5mg / progesterone 100mg per cap)
- Estriol 0,05% vaginal crème 50g tube with applicator - pregnanediol 10mg 60caps (gel-free)
- Pregnanediol 30mg 60caps (gel-free)
- Progesterone 50mg 60 caps
- Progesterone 100mg 60 caps
- Pro Gest Body Cream 60ml tube
- Testosterone 10mg 60 caps
- Androstenadion spray 2,5mg / Spray 60ml

MEDICINES WITH OSTEOPOROSIS

There are various natural products which are well suited as prevention or for the treatment of acute osteoporosis,. We differentiate primarily between homoeopathic and ortho-molecular preparations. The first generally promote – on the energetic- informative level (they are "non-substantial") – the bone and tooth structure of the body. The second furnish the body with the actual minerals and vitamins which are necessary for the generation of bone substance.

It is important, with degenerative bone illnesses, to continue treatment over many years and to have a consistently cow's milk free and/or milk reduced nutrition!

Homeopathic Complex Remedies:

Oss Regen (Pekana): Spagyric / homoeopathic complex remedy from the plant and mineral realms. It is to be used on cases of decreased bone density, inflammations of the periostium, slipped disks, etc.. (Oss rain is freely available in drops 50ml or 100ml).

Osteoheel (Heel): Homoeopathic product from the plant, mineral and animal realms This medicine is suitable for the relief of inflammations of the periostium and other bone illnesses. (Osteoheel is available in tablet form).

Calcium 1 and 2 of (Weleda): Anthroposophical remedy, dynamically treated. Weleda's Calcium 1&2 consists of mineral, animal and vegetable components. This is the only product on the market with two different powders, to be taken one in the morning and the other in the evening, a preparation adapted completely to the body's physical and bio-rhythmical needs! (available as 2x50g, 2x100g or as 500g).

Urticalcin (Bioforce): Homoeopathic product from the plant and mineral realms. Indicated in cases of calcium deficiency symptoms, for the support of the building of bones, fragile fingernails etc.. (available in tablet form).

Equisetum (Cerium): This preparation is optimally suitable to promote and regulate the body's structural and organizing forces. It not only unfolds its effect in the generation of bone structure but it also helps in the cleansing of connective tissue and the promotion of kidney activity. Because of these additional attributes, Equisetum is an ideal parallel medication with each osteoporosis therapy (available as drops)!

Trace elements and vitamins, which promote the body's structural forces:

Kalzium Plus (Burgerstein): This preparation for the preservation of a healthy bone mass also contains further synergistically working mineral substances and trace elements, together with calcium and magnesium, such as: zinc, manganese and copper as well as vitamins C, D3, K, B6 and folic acid.

Dolomite (Burgerstein): Dolomite chewing tablets contain, from a physiological point of view, the ideal combination of 2 parts calcium to 1 part magnesium. It is therefore optimally suitable to supply these minerals, necessary for the generation of bone structure and conservation, to the body, (available as chewing tablets).

All these important vitamins, minerals and natural hormones are available today, in natural and ortho-molecular quality, at the **Paracelsus Clinic Pharmacy.**

Dr. Thomas Rau, M.D.
Paracelsus Klinik Lustmühle,
9062 Lustmühle (bei St.Gallen)
Switzerland

Copyright © 2002 Dr. Thomas Rau
All Rights Reserved

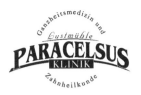

22

Mononucleosis, Glandular Fever (Pfeiffer's Disease) and Epstein Barr Virus

Pfeiffer's disease (= glandular fever = infectious mononucleosis) is, as everybody knows, an acute illness which occurs endemically at regular intervals but also frequently as an epidemic. It affects mostly older children and young adults. It can be transmitted by a high degree of physical contact, less so by airborne droplet infection; therefore this illness is often also called "kissers' disease". This disease manifests itself very typically as severe tonsillitis and is therefore not infrequently mistaken for strepto-angina. But it can also be accompanied by severe enlargement of the lymph nodes, pre-eminently in the neck and imperceptible at the start. Likewise, involvement of the liver and of whole of the lymphatic system is frequently diagnosed. In typical cases the number of monocytes in the blood also increases. An antibody test may be carried out on a tonsil swab.

A typical diagnostic symptom is the lack of response to antibiotics. Characteristically there can also often be a strong blotchy red skin rash (which however disappears within three days) when amino-penicillin is taken: unfortunately this antibiotic is still being prescribed in cases of strepto-angina. The antibiotic treatment of mononucleosis should be regarded as a mistake as this disease is caused by a virus, the Epstein-Barr virus, which like the herpes virus can transform itself into a "slow virus form".

The acute picture of mononucleosis is frequently very conclusive, with a strong feeling of being ill, fever, enormous weakness, sore throat and large tonsils which occasionally become ulcerated on one or both sides. The lymph nodes are always enlarged. The mostly young patients are often in a very weakened state and orthostatically frail for weeks on end, they also frequently complain of stomachache and nausea. On examination you mostly find enlargement of the liver, often splenomegaly (enlargement of the spleen) and large lymph nodes in the groin.

In a typically long and drawn out illness, as a therapist one frequently worries whether it might not in fact be a case of acute leukaemia. In such cases patients are sometimes offered ridiculous diagnoses and advised to visit a specialist. In orthodox medicine there are hardly any effective ways of treating acute mononucleosis. In our opinion any anti-inflammatory or even antibiotic form of treatment furthers the development of the much more complicated chronic form. But effective treatment of the acute form is relatively simple for the doctor who uses isopathic biological methods.

Seen from the point of view of holistic medicine, the chronic picture of the Epstein-Barr virus infection is considerably more radical and more complicated. It is supposed that the virus can transform itself into a slow virus stage and that this occurs during the development of detectable, persistent IgG antibodies, occasionally even IgM, although this is no longer the typical clinical picture; but the disease may present itself quite differently. It is very important that anyone giving holistic treatment should recognise this clinical picture:

- Chronic tiredness, weakness, tendency towards depression, lacki of energy
- A chronic tendency to suffer from headaches, sensitivity to smoke, radiation, and geopathic stress
- Neurological problems such as visual disturbances, inability to concentrate
- Susceptibility to infections

Chronic Epstein-Barr infection is one of the most frequent causes contributing to "chronic fatigue syndrome", mostly in combination with heavy metal contamination and dysbiosis. On the basis of Enderlein's

Table 1: Pfeiffer's disease (glandular fever) – treatment by biological means

Acute phase (as for the majority of acute viral diseases):

Diet:
- No lactoproteins or meat. In adults particularly, restriction of food intake.
- Fruits should be peeled, best steamed; no bananas (thickening of the lymph)
- Vegetables (alkaline), different types of grain, rice, oatmeal broth, avocados
- Liver-and-gall tea, sage tea.

Medications:
- Relivora complex: take 15 drops four to six times daily
- Quentakehl 5X alternating daily with Notakehl 5X: 6 to 8 drops two to three times a day, dropped into the nose or inhaled
- Rebas 4X: twice daily scatter the contents of one capsule into the mouth, and before swallowing mix well with saliva
- Lymphomyosot: take 20 drops four to six times daily
- Where there is swelling of the liver: Mucedokehl 4X: take 1 capsule three times, after seven days take one capsule twice
- Utilin "weak" and Recarcin: take one capsule of each per week
- To revitalise the milieu: take Alkala N: ⁄4 spoonful twice daily, Sanum vitamin B complex and vitamin C 1-3 grams daily, zinc 30 mg daily and selenium 100-200 mcg daily

Supplementary forms of treatment:
- warming baths, bandaging around the liver area, scarf around the neck
- Neural Therapy Bl. 23 (stimulation, warding off stress) and tonsils with Engystol N, Echinacea comp. S ampoule, Tonsilla comp. alternating with Galium heel, procaine 1%
- in serious cases in adults: colonic irrigation, ozone therapy and vitamin C infusion

Table 2: chronic Epstein-Barr syndrome – treatment by biological means

Its development is always caused by a number of factors, the Epstein-Barr virus only contributes to its development. It is important to look for blockades as well as to offer milieu and orthomolecular treatment.

For dental problems and heavy metal intoxication:
- Orthopantogram, DMPS test for Hg, Sn, Pd and copper
- For revitalisation and excretion of heavy metals: Vitamin C: 3 grams daily Selenomethionine: 1-2 daily; zinc tablets (Burgerstein): 2 each evening, possibly DMSA capsules, 2 capsules per week

To support the nerve cells:
- Sanum vitamin B complex: one injection twice a week
- Biofrid plus evening primrose oil: 1 capsule three times daily; alternating on a daily basis with Lipiscor: 5 capsules twice daily
- Wheatgerm oil, cold pressed: take 30 ml daily
- Mapurit: take 1 capsule twice daily

Treatment with Enderlein remedies:
- Mucokehl 3X, Nigersan 3X, Pinikehl 4X suppositories, alternating on a daily basis: use 1 per day, inserted into the rectum
- Quentakehl 5X: introduce 5 to 8 drops into the nose three to four times daily
- Utilin "S" weak: take 1 capsule per week
- Test with Polysan Dx

Supplementary forms of treatment (select one or more):
- Neural therapy: thyroid, suprarenal gland, roof of the throat, tonsils: according to findings
- Medications: Coenzyme comp., Ubichinon comp., Tonsilla comp., Engystol N, Latensin, Viscum forte comp. A

discoveries, only milieu factors are responsible for the fact that these very big Epstein-Barr viruses transform themselves into a slow form. Therefore the problem of this disease can also only be solved by revitalisation of the milieu and the release of blockades in the patient's body. Tables 1 and 2 describe plans for the treatment of acute glandular fever and chronic Epstein-Barr syndrome.

Dr. Thomas Rau, m.d.
Paracelsus Klinik Lustmühle,
9062 Lustmühle (bei St.Gallen)
Switzerland

Lecture given at the 1998 Sanum therapy conference
Published in Sanum Post No. 43 1998
Copyright © 1998 Dr. Thomas Rau
All Rights Reserved

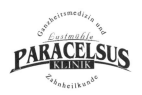

23

Environmental Diseases
Chronic Fatigue Syndrome

ETIOLOGY:
both only explainable with "Barrel-Thinking":
polycausal, both nearly always toxically caused.

Combination frequently:

- leaky gut syndrome (hair mineral analysis)
- trace element dysbalance, low intracellular elements as Manganese, Chromium
- toxic metals, as
  - Aluminium
  - Lead
  - Palladium!!!
  - Copper
  - Mercury!!
  - Root Canal Fillings are very cell-toxic
  - Hyperacidity and mostly Protein excess!
  - Residuals of neurotropic Virus diseases! (EBV, POLIO, Measels)
  - Vaccinations?

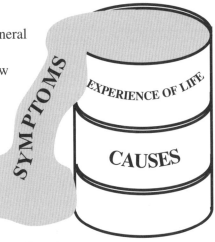

THERAPY: It is justified and important just to treat and detoxify, even when you don't know a single cause.

- EDTA-Infusions, 1–2 x per week: with:
    - Vitamines: Vit. C 7,5 gr, Vitamines B Komplex Vitamine E 200mg
    - Magnesium and Calcium (after EDTA-Infusions) i.V.
    - Ubichinon comp. / Thalamus comp. / Cerebrum comp. /
    - Katalysts of citric acid cycle (once per week one serie)
    - H_2O_2 (3%),carefully rising dose, beginning with 1 ml, up to 10 ml
    - Procain carefully rising in dosage, beginning with 1 ml, up to 5 ml.
- Homeopathic drops, with Nosodes of all tested nosodes, mostly containing insectizydes (Lindan, etc.), former vaccination virusus, Arsenicum album comp. (Pascoe), glioma injeel, Hepar comp., Lymphomyosot
- Orally: Alkala N, Antioxydants, EPA and EPO unsaturated fatty acids. / Vit B Komplex.
- MOST IMPORTANT: Tooth detoxification / All root canals out!! Mercury, tin and palladium detoxification!!!

TREATMENT LASTS AT LEAST 6 MONTHS!

Dr. Thomas Rau, M.D.
Paracelsus Klinik Lustmühle,
9062 Lustmühle (bei St.Gallen)
Switzerland

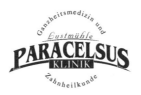

24

The causes of epilepsy
from a holistic point of view

In epilepsy potentials of the central nervous system are released in batches in large quantities: these can lead to convulsions but also to small eruptions and failures of the motor system or sensory nerves. According to whereabouts in the brain the potentials are released, other symptoms apart from convulsions can also occur, e.g. personality changes, small jerking movements, shooting headaches, but also losses of function such as visual disturbances or paralysis, etc. Very similar changes can also be seen typically on an EEG during an acute attack of migraine. In any case it is a fact that in epileptics excessive and uncontrollable nerve potentials are released and can make an impact.

From the holistic point of view there are two possibilities:

➤ the stimulus threshold of the nerve cells is lowered, and therefore even small electrical potentials can have an effect in the brain, or

➤ there are failures which release electrical potentials which are absorbed by the cerebral nerves or cause disruption in the brain.

Orthodox medicine takes note of the fact that pathological potentials exist, and these are suppressed by strong medication (anti-epileptic drugs). The normal nerve cell functions are also suppressed and this can lead to restrictions of the cerebral function at other levels, e.g. fatigue, inability to concentrate, inability to co-ordinate, personality changes, stupor.

But another grave problem is the side-effects on the metabolism of the anti-epileptic drugs which can occur mostly as a form of cell metabolism: gingival accretions (Tegretol), disorders of the cells of the liver (Depakine/Tegretol) or haemopoietic disorders.

The causes

Attempts have been made from a holistic point of view to identify the causes of the abnormal potentials, which are mostly caused by a number of factors:

- Lowering of the stimulus threshold:
- – Lack of trace elements:

Certain trace elements and minerals stabilise the nerve cells: magnesium, zinc, manganese and others. Sometimes these materials can show up in the blood or urine, sometimes in mineral analysis of the hair. Often intensive treatment with doses of trace elements can have a very positive effect in reducing the frequency of the convulsions.

- – Lack of vitamins:

The effect of certain vitamins is to stabilise the cell membranes, but epileptics frequently have a very low level of these: Vitamin E and Vitamin B, also small amounts of folic acid. The level of the individual vitamins can be ascertained in laboratory tests.

- – Heavy metals:

Metals (mercury, palladium, tin, lead, copper), which are mostly to be found in tooth fillings, are absorbed by the body and stored in the nerve cells, the brain and the neuroganglions. They are the opponents of the trace elements mentioned above (manganese, selenium, magnesium, etc) and as a result lower the nerve stimulus threshold.

– Toxic products:

Most epileptics have hidden disorders of the intestine and changes to their intestinal flora. It becomes possible for bacterial poisons to form, and these are also absorbed. Materials which are toxic to the membranes and cells can also cause irritation. Bowel activity can be considerably improved by discovering food allergies, treating bacterial infestations and making changes to the permeability of the intestine, and as a result the toxic load on the body can be reduced.

The diet which we recommend to epileptics on an individual basis takes account of these contexts and also of the need for large amounts of vitamins and trace elements (the diet is to be found in the article "Holistic medical investigations and the treatment of epilepsy" in SANUM-Post 57). However, it consistently avoids food allergens and all types of food which contain preservatives (E numbers) as well as well-fried and well-grilled food, as these contain products of cellular decay, modified fats and so-called free radicals. It is interesting that epileptics are almost always found to be allergic to cow's milk products. This can then lead to strain on the lymphatic system, a reduction in cell respiration and again, as described above, to metabolic overload of the tissues.

– Alcohol and other toxic foodstuffs, nicotine:

Alcohol, but also preservatives and phosphates used as food stabilisers, can modify nerve cell activity and cause excitation of the cerebral nerves.

– Fatigue:

If the body is overtired, products of the metabolism become modified and are no longer completely processed, the excretion of melatonin is modified and there can be powerful disturbances to the nerves.

– Changes to the acid-base balance, excess of acid:

The greater the excess of acid in a patient's tissues, the more heavy metals can be released and affect them, the less oxygen is absorbed by the tissues and the less toxic products are excreted. However, excess of acid in the tissues also involves changes to the pH value of the intercellular space through which all catabolic products from the cells and toxins are transported away and through which the cells are provided with nutrients.

It has been possible to prove scientifically (spectroanalysis and electron microscope investigations by Prof. Hartmut Heine) that polysaccharide molecules with a high molecular weight form a thick, directional network in the interstitial space (intercellular space) along which materials move. If the tissues are very acid, H+ ions (acid ions) are given off into the intercellular fluid and lead to a needled felt-like cross-linking of these polysaccharide molecules so that it is no longer possible for things to pass or be transported through the interstitial space. The result is then an increase in the level of poisoning of the tissues and cells and a reduction in "cell respiration", as the supply of oxygen is also affected. The result of cell metabolism with insufficient oxygen is an increase in the fermentation of the cells in order to provide energy and an increase in lactose (lactic acid), which again is acidic. Excess of acid, to a great extent caused by diet, is therefore an important factor in maintaining epilepsy and one which works on different levels.

Excess of acid can be treated most sustainably through diet, but also by prescribing alkaline remedies such as ALKALA N and ALKALA T. Nowadays it can be proved very easily that an organism contains excess acid by measuring the pH value, the electrical resistance value and the redox potential of the lymph (represented by saliva), blood and urine. This test is called "bioterrain analysis" (cf. BTA apparatus made by the Vega family) and is carried out in modern biological doctors' practices such as the Lustmühle Paracelsus Clinic.

- Increased levels of non-neural stimulation factors (strengthening of electrical potential by external factors):

- Galvanic currents from dental materials:

Like a battery, the metals in mixed alloys (e.g. nickel, mercury and copper) from tooth replacement materials can release galvanic current potentials which can be measured in milliamps. These exceed the normal nerve potentials by a factor of 1,000 to 100,000! In this way currents can be released which the brain registers and converts in terms of epileptic potentials. A similar effect comes from metal parts from the post used to support a crown, even X-ray-proof root filling materials, which often contain metal ions. Again and again we see root canal fillings as the cause of epileptic fits, often beginning even months or years after root fillings have been started, as they can often be tolerated for a very long time.

In children we frequently see that epilepsy can become more intense or even be triggered following the use of dental braces, particularly because of the clamps which fix them to the teeth. It is the solder in particular, often containing cadmium or lead, which releases galvanic currents.

The measurement of galvanic currents in the mouth can be carried out very easily using an ammeter and a voltometer (e.g. galvanometer in the Vega test apparatus).

Electromagnetic and electrostatic fields in the bedroom can also lead to enormous stress and raising of the endogenic neural potentials, particularly during the night. Similarly, an increase in stress can also cause this type of field as a result of working at a computer monitor (the modern LCD flat screens are much better in this respect).

Electromagnetic stresses, and also so-called "geopathic" stresses (in common parlance wrongly named "water courses"), cause a change not only in the measurable nerve cell potential but also in the vegetative nerve cell function (sympathetic and parasympathetic) which control the ground potential of the organism. Thus in epileptics one very frequently sees a sympathetic nervous system potential which is raised by a large amount – that is, a basic tonus caused by stress – which also explains the susceptibility of epileptics to additional stress.

Nowadays this potential too can be measured objectively by progressive biological physicians using ANSA (Autonomous Nerve System Analysis or heart rate variability test), which measures the important interplay between the tonicity and the body's ability to ability to relax. Patients with epileptic fits often display bizarrely reduced parasympathetic abilities.

–   Dental foci of interference, impacted wisdom teeth and dental root fillings, localised irritation by toxins:

In every dead tooth, even in root canal treatment which is carried out "properly", there are highly toxic proteins from dead bodies and free radicals (thioether, mercaptane, indole, catole, even formaldehyde). At a local level these can react chemically or with the nerves or can interfere with the interstitial system. Therefore one should always look for dead teeth and both bacterial and chemical interference factors in all patients who suffer epileptic fits.

Impacted wisdom teeth have a particularly energetic connection with the cerebrum and a tendency to convulsions. Therefore, when epileptic fits start to happen in adolescents and young adults, one should always consider that the predispositions of the wisdom teeth might be wrong. The biochemical and physical mechanism of these interrelationships has unfortunately not yet been discovered. It has however been proven that along the course of the meridians (paths of reduced electrical resistance) there is a change in the membrane potentials.

- Mechanical, infectious and post-traumatic causes:

Orthodox medicine also recognises that the formation of scar tissue in the brain, high pressure in the brain and inflammation can change the potentials of the electric currents in the brain as a result of localised irritation. Viral inflammations can cause localised swelling and thus cause irritation, but this can also be caused by the products of cell decomposition.

But too little notice is taken of the chronic viral stresses which we find again and again, whether these conditions arise from obvious or from viral infections of the brain (neurotropic viruses) which have occurred unnoticed in the past: herpes simplex, herpes zoster, cytomegalus, parotitis virus, poliomyelitis and also, among others, the measles virus.

It is particularly worth noticing the immunisation viruses which are wrongly regarded as not harmful but can cause a chronic underlying viral infection: immunisations against infantile paralysis, measles, tick-borne encephalitis and even hepatitis B – the widespread use of which is being recommended by all and sundry!

Very many of these viral stresses and viral diseases caught later can be proved today by means of blood tests for IgG and IgM (immuno-globulins) and even recently by means of the direct proof of the presence of the virus, the PCR (polymer chain reaction).

The treatment of these stresses must then of course be carried out very specifically using nosode remedies and cytokines, which is the job of the holistic physician with experience of these things.

In practically all "epilepsy patients" it is possible to find a mixture of different causes and to achieve significant improvement by dealing with all these factors. In most cases anti-epileptic drugs are no longer needed after a few months or only in low doses. The stability of the neural potential is improved, the frequency of fits is reduced or they stop completely. The pathological electrical potentials in the EEG (brain current graph) very frequently disappear within 6 – 12 months.

Readers may have noticed in the above models that I mostly refer to "patients with epileptic fits" or that the word "epilepsy" is in quotation marks. This is because patients of this type are very often labelled as "epileptics" at an early stage and this to the layperson is irrevocable and is linked with ideas of a reduction in mental capacity. According to our experiences this is just not justified if the patient is treated holistically. When the above-named factors are treated consistently, patients mostly find that their fits stop and their neurological and cerebral symptoms disappear – these often being made worse by anti-epileptic drugs and just being another form of expression of their toxic or other stresses.

Examples

At this point let us look at two examples of typical patients:

O.E., 14-year-old boy:

Was brought for examination after getting strong side-effects from anti-epileptic drugs: dysfunction of his sense of taste, fatigue, lack of interest, a drop-off in his performance at school, putting on weight, an increasingly phlegmatic personality, dropping out into "bad company". The boy is the son of a single mother who was clearly under a lot of pressure. Very fast growth-rate in the past two years, fast approaching puberty. An unhealthy diet, sweets, a lot of sausage, sweetened drinks, almost a litre of milk a day because this is "so healthy". A regular diet of television! His first grand mal fit happened as the result of a "taster" work placement involving physical work, which was then followed by others, in the beginning even while he was receiving treatment for epilepsy. The first EEG showed a temporo-occipital obstruction on the right, then later generalised epileptic potentials. An MRI scan (Magnetic Resonance Imaging: computer tomography of the brain) showed no unusual features. Treatment with Lamictal, in the early stages even with phenobarbital!

The holistic examination showed a pasty habitus, thick tongue, pale skin with a lot of water retention, a rather cold, calcium carbonicum constitution. Darkfield microscopy of the live blood showed completely rigid leucocytes, signs of blood alkalinity, otherwise no particularly significant findings. The thermoregulation diagnosis showed definite signs of intolerance of certain foodstuffs, with strong lymphatic irritation and "cold" blocking of the points of the small intestine. Teeth normal. Noticeably hyper-reactive heart points!

Comments, procedure and course of treatment:
The pasty calcium-carbonicum constitution linked with the classic thermography findings made one think of deposits of morbid matter on the mesenchyme accompanied by toxic stress. The main treatment therefore consisted of detoxification, support of the liver metabolism and diet. To start treatment: building up of the intestinal flora using isopathic products from the SANUM company, building up of the enteral immune system with the Peyer's patches (REBAS 4X capsules). A strict diet without cow's milk, with little meat, no more sausages, no acid-forming sweetened drinks.

Acid links together the mesenchymal polysaccharide network and prevents detoxification. Therefore in addition a course of basic (alkaline) therapy with ALKALA N and minerals (multi-mineral tablets from the Burgerstein company). No neurotropic cerebral viruses were found. The dental panoramic picture showed that all his wisdom teeth were developing very actively. This raises the disposition towards fits very considerably, which is also why puberty is a time when children have a greater tendency to convulsions. Therefore also magnesium therapy and MUCOKEHL, two remedies which we allocate to the cardiac function circulation. Homeopathic calcium carbonicum 200X once a week.

The treatment went very well: the patient was very co-operative because previously he had suffered as a result of his own personality changes and being a social outcast. He kept strictly to the vegetarian diet, carried out his deacidification programme and took the medications. He remained free of fits despite stopping his anti-epileptic treatment completely within 6 weeks! In the meantime the patient has been free of antiepileptic drugs for 6 months and is still in good health. His school performance is better than it had been previously.

Here the causes were a combination of toxicity of the tissues, caused by the intestine, and an increased tendency to fits because of hormone changes and decreased resorption of trace elements, also caused by the intestine. The electromagnetic stress from the television was probably a concomitant factor.

> Never forget: in the case of epileptics always think of the wisdom teeth, lack of trace elements, heavy metal overloads and enterotoxicity!

Ch.F., a 48-year-old American woman:

A gracile patient, in need of care, with spastic tetraplegic paralysis, had been putting on weight for years, with generalised epileptic fits, resistant to treatment despite taking a variety of anti-epileptic medications. A physical examination showed nothing definite. Her regulation thermography was typical, with thermographically over-regulating results for the small intestine. The dental X-ray showed an impacted wisdom tooth and a wisdom tooth socket in the left lower jaw remaining after an extraction, but with a small piece of the root bone left in the socket very close to the mandibularis nerve.

Only after questioning did the relatives confirm that the fits had become more frequent in the period following the removal of that wisdom tooth. The normal initial therapy described below brought about no change, but the milk-free, mild, allergen-free diet according to Dr Rau, designed to protect the small intestine, improved her feeling of wellbeing.

The significant change of mood came about with the dental treatment. Despite an increase in the number of epileptic fits, the impacted wisdom tooth on the right lower jaw was removed first. From this point in time onwards the patient had a different kind of fit: petit mal instead of the previous generalised fits which had focused on the right side.

With the surgical removal of the old root from the impacted wisdom tooth, extracting it from a gelose cartliagineous material, and very careful release of the mandibularis nerve, the patient once again had a big fit during the operation, with spontaneous micturation. This was her last fit!

From this intervention onwards, the patient had no more fits. During the course of treatment she was slowly weaned off the anti-epileptic medications within a few weeks. The spasticity slowly disappeared, and the patient made an enormous recovery emotionally and cognitively,

Disrupted wisdom teeth lead to obstructions of the small intestine / cardiac circulatory system and influence the patient's general tendency to fit and emotional stability.

In all problems with the cardiac and small intestine function circulation always think of wisdom teeth, also in cases of epilepsy and cyclothymia (manic-depressive reactions).

Dr. Thomas Rau, M.D.
Medical Director
Paracelsus Klinik Lustmühle,
9062 Lustmühle (bei St.Gallen)
Switzerland

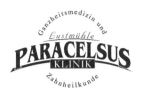

25

Epilepsy: Medical investigation and Biological Treatment

The first part of this two-part series of articles on the natural healing aspects of epilepsy, in SANUM Post No. 56, dealt with the causes from a holistic point of view. This second part now deals with the treatment of the illness.

First I shall list and explain the typical diagnostic findings of the toxic and/or lymphatic stresses.

In our clinic the following investigations are normally carried out at the start of therapy:

- Clinical physical examination

The tongue, the periodontium (gums), lymph nodes, skin tone, iris, liver, spleen and anus are examined. In accordance with the criteria of Chinese medicine, this physical examination gives the experienced biological physician very many clues as to blockages, congestion or overload of the liver and intestines. From this one can discover the level of lymphatic toxicity and also find clues as to the intactness or otherwise of the intestinal system.

- Orthopantomograph (OPG)

(a dental X-ray) pinpoints root spikes and deep fillings as well as impacted wisdom teeth or other points of interference in the jaw area.

- Testing for heavy metals by means of the intravenous DMPS test

shows the presence of metals and the excretion of them in the urine:

mercury, tin and silver from amalgam fillings, palladium and copper from gold fillings, nickel and possibly also arsenic/lead/cadmium from solder.

- Measurement of galvanic currents in and around the mouth

is a very simple investigation which could be carried out by every doctor in his/her practice. It shows the release of ions and the way the teeth work like a battery. This is a part of the clinical examination of each patient.

- ANSA (heart rate variability test or "rhythmogram")

shows any blocking of the vegetative nervous system, mostly an accompanying cause of toxic overload of the organism.

- Darkfield microscopy of the vital blood

is an extremely revealing investigation which shows the toxic stress on an organism, the presence of the wrong milieu and excess of acid. Excess acid is namely one of the important causes of reduction in the stimulus potential.

- Assessment of the amount of excess acidity and of mineral content

Bioterrain analysis (BTA) and measurements of the pH of the urine.

- Hair mineral analysis

on the one hand shows toxic overload, on the other hand gives important pointers to defective bowel function and increased permeability of the intestinal system (leaky gut syndrome). It is interesting that high values for aluminium are very frequently found in patients with a tendency to convulsions, which is a symptom of excess acid in the tissues and of the leaky gut.

- Possibly thermoregulation diagnosis

to ascertain whether there are any food allergies and missing colonies of bacteria in the intestine, but also to assess the significance of dental interferences and heavy metal overloads, which give a typical profile in thermoregulation diagnosis.

THE BIOLOGICAL TREATMENT OF EPILEPSY

First and foremost the stress situation must be improved, using the approaches named above. As a result of this, the tendency towards epilepsy is mostly improved in the long term to the point where there are hardly any or no further attacks. However, this mostly takes several months, during which time other treatment consisting mainly of chemical medication can be slowly reduced.

This reduction does however mostly really only bear fruit if at the same time treatment is carried out which consists of biological medication and diet.

The treatment includes various approaches:

Every part of the therapy is addressed separately below. The biological treatment of epilepsy and tendency to convulsions leads to a considerable improvement in mental activity, alertness and general well-being.

- Diet
- Intestinal cleansing
- Orthomolecular therapy
- Detoxification therapy (heavy metals, toxins in the liver and intestine)
- Removal of foci of interference
- Lifestyle
- Improvement of the brain cell metabolism

Diet

On the one hand, the diet should re-tune the metabolism and protect the intestinal mucous membrane. This is done by avoiding the usual intestinal allergens, which consist mostly of the following:

- cow's milk products
- irritant citrus fruits such as oranges, kiwis, mandarins and citrus juice
- pork and pork products.

On the other hand the diet should be alkaline, it should contain a lot of minerals and lead to removal of excess acid. Care should be taken to include polyunsaturated fatty acids, also glutamic acid, choline, also B-vitamins, antioxidants such as Vitamins C and E, beta-carotene, octocosanol, e.g. from wheatgerm oil, alfalfa sprouts (lucerne) and bamboo shoots. Choline is contained in lecithin, fish, wheatgerm, wheat products and soya; tyrosine in bananas, yeast, avocado and fish. The following foodstuffs have proved very valuable:

- all vegetables (preferably lightly steamed, as if eaten raw frequently they cannot be broken down because of weakness of the pancreas, then they begin to ferment)
- cereal products, also egg-free dough products (durum wheat dough products = Italian pasta)
- potatoes and chestnuts (very alkaline), e.g. potatoes boiled in their skins, then peeled, are ideal in the evening
- meat: only poultry or fish, but each only once or twice a week! The avoidance of animal protein is possibly the most important thing in the alkaline re-tuning of the metabolism and intestinal flora!
- fruit (all fruits only to be eaten in the morning; no citrus fruits).

This diet must be followed for a period of several months!

Intestinal cleansing:
Cleansing of the intestine is already principally guaranteed by the diet, as this re-tunes and renews the intestinal flora. The patient should gradually accustom him-/herself to increasing amounts of raw food including carrots, fennel, celery/celeriac, but everything finely grated. At the start of treatment colonic irrigation has proved very beneficial: this should be combined with deep, soft massage of the bowel to stimulate the vagal system. Have lots of warm drinks, e.g. fennel tea, peppermint tea.

The actual building up of the intestinal flora and intestinal mucous membrane is recommended as follows:

Building up the intestinal flora (according to Dr Thomas Rau, MD)

To build up the intestinal mucous membrane:

- Mucosa comp. Amp. (Heel): one ampoule twice daily,
  to be injected at the M25 point or drunk.
- Diet according to Dr Werthmann

Regulation of the intestinal flora:

- At the start: FORTAKEHL 5X: 1 tablet 3 times,
- then PEFRAKEHL 4X capsules or 5X drops: for 2 weeks,
- then SANKOMBI 5X drops: 2 times 10 drops, or MUCOKEHL
  5X and NIGERSAN 5X.

Immune stimulation:

- UTILIN and RECARCIN capsules: one of each per week
- REBAS 4X capsules: 1 capsule twice daily
- PROPIONIBACTERIUM AVIDUM 5X capsules: 1–2 per week.

Orthomolecular therapy:

- Magnesium in combination with vitamin E: MAPURIT: 2 times 1
  capsule, or magnesium orotate (Burgerstein): 2 times one tablet
  and Vitamin E (Burgerstein): 400 mg daily. Magnesium raises the
  stimulus and depolarisation threshold, vitamin E stabilises the
  nerve cell membrane. Orotic acid supports the intake of acid by the
  cells.
- Vitamin B complex (Burgerstein): 2 times 1 tablet
- Vitamin C 1000 mg (Burgerstein) tablets: 1–2 tablets daily
- Zinc tablets (Burgerstein): 1 tablet (30 mg) in the evening, but
  intermittently
- Manganese (contained in Anti-Ox/De-Tox from Burgerstein): 1
  tablet, 10–20 mg, twice daily; stabilises the cell membranes and
  reduces the number of fits
- Taurine: 0.5 to 2 g daily also reduces the number of fits. (Taurine
  is also recommended in cases of heavy metal poisoning, from
  which epileptics often suffer in any case; also methionine)
- Selenium: 100 mg daily

- Dimethylglycine: 100–200 mg; this is a preliminary stage of the amino acid glycine which has a calming effect on the brain and reduces the frequency of convulsions.

Caveat: Aspartame, the artificial sweetener, which is contained in almost all "diet" drinks, can cause epileptic fits particularly in children!

Aspartame is forbidden to epileptics! Take similar care with folic acid and high doses of Omega 3 fatty acids. They can also cause fits.

Metals including aluminium, cadmium, mercury and lead support frequent fitting.

Detoxification therapy, heavy metals, intestinal toxins

Heavy metals are very frequently the cause of epilepsy and must be looked for as a matter of routine: hair mineral analysis, DMPS test of the urine.

Mostly it is a matter of mercury, palladium, tin, all from dental fillings, then aluminium (including in children) and lead.

For detoxification one needs antagonists, mostly selenium, zinc, vitamins (see too the article on excretion "The SANUM excretion cure" in SANUM Post No.55, 2001)

Important: no clarification and treatment of epileptics without a strict search for heavy metals, dental clarification, dental galvanic currents and root toxins from root fillings.

Intestinal toxins are caused by faulty intestinal flora, often following a course of antibiotic treatment and, among other things, when the diet is faulty. Colonic irrigation, building up the intestinal flora and diet are the most important approaches to treatment.

Because of the enterohepatic circulation, the liver is the first point at which the intestinal toxins collect and is often enormously overloaded, whether with the products of fermentation or with free radicals from the metabolism of bacteria. These patients often feel a non-specific pressure in the upper abdomen or are restless for 1–3 hours at night in the "liver period". As a result a course of liver treatment is often necessary:

A possible course of therapy to support the liver:

- Liv 52 Ayurmedica: 3 times 1 to 3 times 2 tablets
- Carduus marianus Ceres drops: 5 drops 3 times daily (supports detoxification of the cells)
- VIT. B COMPLEX SANUM N: 2 times 1 ampoule; Taraxum (Ceres): 3 times 5 tablets (supports the flow of gall)
- MUSCARSAN 6X: 5 drops 1–3 times daily (supports detoxification of the cells, removing organic liver toxins).

Removal of foci of interference:

This is the classic form of therapy of the biological physician: the foci of interference are looked for using dental X-rays, investigation of thermoregulation, possibly also electro-acupuncture, then treated in a targeted manner by means of neural therapy. The foci of interference most frequently found in epileptics are: dental foci, root-treated teeth, dental braces in children, tonsillar foci, also old scar tissue, old gynaecological foci, the intestine as a "focus of interference".

Lifestyle:

A well-regulated day is extremely important: regular intake of food, chewed well, stick to drinks between mealtimes and in large quantities, teas to cleanse the blood, no sweetened drinks; children should not drink iced drinks.

Some physical activity each day, but no great exertion! Walking, hiking, gardening, etc. are very good; cycling. No extreme exposure to the sun – wear protection against the sun's rays. Regular times for sleep!

For children: no television and no computer games. The small screens on games of dexterity are particularly bad!

Improvement of the brain cell metabolism:

Isopathic remedies: Prof. Enderlein's theory explains to us that the inner and cellular milieu can be influenced by isopathic remedies which are normally present as protein molecules in the cells. They alter the viscosity of the bodily and cell fluids, thereby enabling detoxification to take place, as well as enabling the intake of nutrients and oxygen by the cells.

Therefore an accompanying course of isopathic treatment should be carried out for epileptics, as well as for all patients with neurological, cognitive and degenerative cerebral problems:

- MUCOKEHL 5X tablets: one tablet in the morning
- NIGERSAN 5X tablets: one tablet in the evening
- ALKALA N base salt: 1 measuring spoonful in water at about 10.00 am and possible also at about 4.00 in the afternoon.

For children: SANKOMBI 5X drops: 8 drops twice daily in the nose for 1–2 years!

Catalysts and similar substances: The energy metabolism of the cells depends on metabolic processes which need enzymes, catalysts and trace elements in order to function. Some of these have already been mentioned under orthomolecular therapies:

- Coenzym Q10 (Burgerstein): 1 tablet twice
- Coenzyme comp. Amp. (Heel): 2 per week, injected or sniffed up the nose.
- Ubichinon com. Amp. (Heel): idem
- CITROKEHL: 5–10 drops three times
- SANUVIS: 60 drops three times
- FORMASAN: 60 drops three times
- ATP Injeel (Heel): one to 3 ampoules per week, injected.

Catalysts from the citric acid cycle (Heel): one ampoule combination of 10 ampoules, of which each ampoule should be given daily by injection (or, for children, sniffed up the nose) in the correct order.

All these catalytic medications have a good stimulant effect on the brain and are an important part of the treatment of chronic neurological diseases. They should be given over a long term, but can also be alternated.

PROPIONIBACTERIUM AVIDUM, the strongest immune stimulant of the SANUM immune biological medicines, also leads to improvement of the cell metabolism in the brain and nerve cells. It is also very effective in slight cerebral dysfunction in old people and children, as well as in migraine. Take 1–2 capsules per week.

The treatment of epilepsy is undertaken on an individual basis according to the findings of regulation medicine. In the summary described above it may appear difficult. But it has the great advantage that it can lead to healing of the problem and improvement of mental alertness! Mostly it consists of prescribing trace elements, detoxifying substances and specific advice on diet and change of diet.

The course of treatment can last for several months, but leads in very many cases to healing of the disease as its causes are removed.

Dr. Thomas Rau, M.D.
Paracelsus Klinik Lustmühle,
9062 Lustmühle (bei St.Gallen)
Switzerland

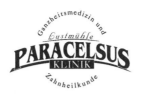

26

Multiple Sclerosis:
Explanations for patients on biological clearing and therapy

Introduction

Thank you for coming to us for clarification and treatment for your suspected, or already diagnosed, M.S. Here we can offer you a really broad perspective and new ways of looking at your illness!. For us M.S. is not just an illness, applied to you like a stamp, without prospect of improvement. We treat our M.S. patients very individually and each one has a different therapy. We do not know the origin of this disease either, but we do know several possible partial causes, which encourage the breakdown of the myelin sheath of the nerve fibres and which we try to exclude one by one. We have achieved very good results this way, among our current long term patients there have been only isolated relapses, which apart from one or two were completely cured.

In general, in subjective terms, the patients do very well in biological therapy and they feel much stronger. We have been able to offer many female patients a considerable improvement in their weakness or even relapses! The disease can be completely cured or go into remission, when we proceed according to the following principles:

PRINCIPLES

1) Principle of constant renewal / Supporting the restorative forces:

All tissues in the human body renew themselves constantly, even nerve sheaths. The renewal processes in the nerve tissues are very slow however and depend on very good "nutrition" for the newly forming fibres. The myelin sheaths destroyed in M.S. largely consist of high grade fats. So if we want to boost their restoration, we need high grade fats (unsaturated fats of vegetable origin, particularly linseed oil, which is rich in omega-6 fatty acids), but also vitamins and high grade essential amino acids such as e.g. lysine, taurine, methionine etc. The so-called "orthomolecular medicine" (specific nutrient replacement) is therefore highly significant. There are also specific „restorative hormones" which we administer individually in the natural form, in order to reinforce the general restorative forces.

2) Eliminating toxic factors:

Present-day nutrition and the environment are very high in preservatives and insecticides, but also in solvents and acids. Some of these have fat-dissolving effects, others however have nerve-damaging effects (insecticides are neurotoxins). But there are also tissue-damaging organic substances in the body, which can likewise destroy nerve substances and also trigger local inflammations, such as e.g. the so-called free radicals from the endogenous metabolism and from toxic bacteria and parasites. Such toxins can be directly eliminated, on the one hand through specific intestinal treatments and the boosting of the intestinal flora, on the other hand with algae therapy (spirulina) as algae have a high capacity for binding toxins. In addition however the liver is also specifically supported in its function of processing organic toxins: with homeopathic stimulation but also with trace elements and amino acids such as e.g. glutamine, and chelate infusions (ion exchange technique).

Ptomaines from root-treated teeth can have a particularly disastrous effect: thio-ether, aldehyde, skatole, which act as highly effective neurotoxins. Professor Haley of the University of Lexington KY/USA has demonstrated that in the destroyed myelin sheaths of M.S. patients there were the same toxins as in the root-treated teeth of these patients. A complete dental rehabilitation and detoxification is therefore extremely important in the treatment of M.S. and in our experience has brought many M.S. patients a significant improvement

Low grade fats, both endogenous and those supplied from outside the body can also have a similarly damaging effect, reinforcing the general inflammatory tendency. The formation of arachidonic acid is increased and this raises the levels of prostaglandins, which can contribute to the destruction of the myelin sheaths. Fried fats are tremendously detrimental, particularly those of animal origin. But also hardened fats and linoleic acid, such as those found in processed foods (margarine, roasted peanuts (!), crisps etc.) are bad! Fats can oxidise in the body, become „rancid" and cause damage. One can prevent this process by ingesting large quantities of antioxidants: selenium, vitamins C and B6, but also B12, beta-carotene and vitamin E. This antioxidant therapy is an important component of our therapy schedule and is initially usually administered by infusion. It is often impressive how much better the patients feel as a result!

Nutrition is an important factor: the diet has to be adjusted to the individual but should contain no fried animal fats and a lot of high grade vegetable fats, but also raw food, sprouting plants, lots of vegetables and no cows milk products, or only very few.

3) Eliminating concomitant infectious factors or autoimmune factors:

As far as we know today, M.S. is not an infectious or viral disease. However in many cases we see that viral influences or stresses can cause an interaction. There are so-called "neurotropic" and "lymphotropic" viruses, which we find in strangely accumulated clusters in M.S. These are among others cytomegaloviruses, herpes simplex and shingles, hepatitis B and also vaccination viruses. We always treat them with Nosodene (rising dilution concentrations of antibodies, which stimulate the immune system to work against them), after which we observe a drop in the concentrations of antibodies, often in parallel with an improvement in the disease.

The therapy recommended in medical school is also based on this, using interferon, a substance which can have an antiviral effect by stimulating the white blood corpuscles. But we find that the doses used in this therapy are too high and lead to too many side effects with only questionable effect. However if the patient is already on Interferon and does not dare to give it up, he or she should still carry out our therapies.

On the basis of very recent studies, it has also been postulated that bacteria which are altered by antibiotic therapies (having no cell wall) or even bacterial components can have a damaging effect on the nerve cells and above all on the lymphocytes. These tissue-penetrating "amoeba-like" elements are no longer correctly recognised by the immune system and invoke autoimmune reactions. A new form of immunological therapy marks these substances and forms with no cell wall and renders them recognisable to the macrophages (feeder cells). This is the modern immunological hapten therapy.

The M.S. Therapy of the Paracelsus Klinik comprises an increasing number of steps and is highly individualised:
- **Antioxidant infusions,** initially usually in infusions to stabilise the situation, subsequently oral (in tablet form)
- **Elimination of heavy metals and organic toxins,** which is initially run in parallel with the infusions but also then accompanies other additional therapies such as cupping massage, colonic hydrotherapies, algae therapies, amino-acid administration etc.
- **Nutritional advice and rehabilitation**
- **Complete dental rehabilitation**
- **Specific administration of natural, anabolising substances, vitamins, unsaturated fatty acids etc.,** to rebuild the nerve substances
- **Acetylcholine** (the transmitter substance for the nerve synapses) in injections or infusions, for hypotonic (slack) paralysis and failures.
- **Immunobiological measures and hapten therapies.**
- **Accompanying measures such as deep infrared saunas** (strong detoxification for toxic substances from the subcutaneous fatty tissue), **local pulsing magnetic field therapy** (boosts cell regeneration and improves the cell membrane potential)

This is a long term therapy over 1 to 2 years, which is however only intensive in the beginning and requires frequent visits to us or the patient's own doctor, where the latter is prepared to administer the infusions according to our directions. Later the therapy is quite simple and can easily be carried out at home. But: there is no M.S. therapy without detoxification from heavy metals and dental toxins, which evidence has shown to be one of the main causes of M.S.!! In the meantime our results with over 70 M.S.-patients have been very good, even when observed for many years. So we are delighted that you too want to come to us for treatment!

On behalf of the whole team of the Paracelsus Klinik in Lustmühle – Al Ronc/Castaneda

Dr. Thomas Rau, M.D.
Paracelsus Klinik Lustmühle,
9062 Lustmühle (bei St.Gallen)
Switzerland

Lecture given at the 1998 Sanum therapy conference
Published in Sanum Post No. 43 1998
Copyright © 1998 Dr. Thomas Rau
All Rights Reserved

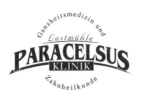

27

Treating the "hyperactive" Child: Causally Oriented Biological Therapy

The number of children, including school-age children, who, driven by inner compulsion, exhibit "hyperactive" behavior, is not small and seems to be on the rise. This pathological behavior is stressful not just for the children, but also for parents, teachers, siblings and of course anyone in their vicinity. Factors such as poor dietary habits have long been under suspicion as the cause of this symptomatology, in which artificial ingredients, such as are found in many "refreshing" soft drinks, are being viewed critically. In addition, other triggering factors have been discussed, such as watching TV for hours every day, which is (no doubt justifiably) considered to be "jointly responsible".

Defining the Hyperactive Syndrome
Unfortunately, the diagnosis to this symptomatology often is still applied to children whose behavior does not fully match up with the actual prerequisites or characteristics of this symptomatology. These prerequisites or characteristics are:

- Early onset of behavioral disorder before the age of five;
- Overactive immoderate behavior appears in conjunction with marked in-attentiveness and lack of perseverance in performing assigned tasks;
- Behavioral disorder is situation-dependent but consistent over the longer term;
- Behavioral disorder includes disturbed social behavior;

- Learning disorders can also be present as well; on the other hand, intelligence disorders tend to be the exception.

Treating the hyperactive child by means of regulative medicine promises good results, because the causes of the disorder are thereby addressed. These causes should be viewed above all as an internal "milieu displacement", and "inner state of disturbance". Contributory factors can include elevated histamine production, trace element and/or vitamin deficiency and heavy metal intoxication – factors capable of lowering the stimulus threshold of nerve cells or the ganglia of the autonomic system.

Thus, there is generally an organic illness associated with any " hyperactive syndrome". It is important to make this clear to the young patient and the parents, since the disorder has usually already been "psychologized". Nevertheless, treatment has to include the entire family, for example with regard to the requirement of a regulated daily activity flow, avoidance of harmful substances and electromagnetic radiation effects (such as the TV set), which can otherwise stress the children. A key part of family-involved therapy likewise includes a dietary plan attuned to the clinical picture.

Treating the Hyperactive Child

Treatment of hyperactive children is long-term and demands a lot of patience, especially from the parents. It is a multifactorial treatment that must be strictly adhered to. The complete therapy of the hyperactive syndrome includes – in addition to diet – intestinal cleansing, diversion (especially in cases involving heavy metal intoxication), orthomolecular therapy, isopathic and immunobiological therapy, and compound homeopathic therapy. Regarding the individual components of the overall therapy, there are some important tips listed below under their keywords. Each therapist will surely incorporate additional treatment steps into the necessary overall therapy, which, for example, can affect the – by no means to be underestimated – elimination and diversion of harmful substances, heavy metals above all.

Intestinal Cleansing

Dietary readjustment to a natural-foods diet as outlined by Dr. Werthmann:

- No eggs or milk or their derivatives, no pork or ham, no anchovies or sardines;
- No canned foods;
- No refined sugar nor products containing refined sugar, especially no carbonated soft drinks such as Coca-Cola, etc.;
- No citrus fruits.

Eating can be spread out over five daily meals, and the atmosphere at mealtimes needs to be calm and relaxed. Foods should also not be heated for too long nor cooked too long in the microwave. Restoration of the intestinal flora by means of milieu therapy, intestinal mucous membrane cleansing and, if needs be, immune-system stimulation:

- Milieu therapy with Pleo™Alkala N and minerals or Alen.
- For intestinal mucous membrane cleansing (besides the Werthmann diet), Mucosa compositum (Heel): drink 1 sip 2x daily or apply at [acupuncture] point M25.
- To promote intestinal flora, begin with Pleo™Fort 5X (1 tablet 3x daily for two weeks), continue with Pleo™Pef 4X (1 capsule Ix daily for two weeks), then Pleo™Sancom or Pleo™Muc 5X with Pleo™Nig 5X (10 drops 2x daily for several months).

Isopathic and Immunobiological Therapy

This therapy should always be combined with orthomolecular therapy. Damage to the intestinal mucous membrane is often accompanied by immune system disorders and susceptibility to infection. Administer the following:

- Pleo™Sancom (8–10 drops 2x daily, preferably inhaled nasally);
- Pleo™Ut N and Pleo™Rec N (rub 1–3 drops into the bend of the elbow 1x daily in alternation);
- Pleo™Alkala N (in the evening, take 1 full measuring spoon dissolved in ½ glass of warm water); see milieu therapy above.

Diversion Therapy

Toxic burdens are quite frequently found in hyperactively disturbed children, particularly in the form of toxic metals such as mercury from amalgam fillings. Often, these harmful metals can be successfully removed with chelating agents. It is also important to know that every harmful metal has an antagonist, with whose help the metal's harmful effects can be neutralized. These antagonists are:

- Calcium, magnesium, vitamin B6, vitamin C for aluminum;
- Selenium, calcium, zinc, chromium, methionine, vitamin C for lead;
- Zinc, selenium, methionine, vitamin C, vitamin B6 for cadmium;
- Selenium, zinc, methionine, cysteine, vitamin C, vitamin E, pectin for mercury. Pleo Chelate taken in drop form is recommended for diversion of toxic heavy metals.

Orthomolecular Therapy

The following agents are indicated for this therapy over a longer period of time:
- Biofrid-Plus capsules in daily alternation with Biofrid salmon-oil capsules (1 capsule 3x daily);
- Multimineral tablets (Burgerstein): 1 tablet daily;
- Pleo™Vit E (1 sip applied Ix weekly);
- Pleo™Vit B Complex (1 sip 2x weekly);
- Mapurit (1 capsule I x daily with liquid).

Compound Homeopathic Therapy

The following agents are indicated for this therapy over the course of several weeks:
- Catalysts of the citric acid cycle (Heel): 1 sip inhaled through the nose every other day, sequence 1 to 10, then a 10-day break, then start over in the same manner,
- On the off days: apply 1 sip of Cerebrum compositum (Heel) alternating with Coenzym compositum (Heel);
- Magnesium phosphoricum 6X or 12X (Schüssler): 3 tablets daily.

With the total therapy outlined here, there is a chance of successfully treatment even the more difficult cases of hyperactive syndrome in children, and at least of achieving distinct improvement.

Dr. Thomas Rau, M.D.
Paracelsus Klinik Lustmühle,
9062 Lustmühle (bei St.Gallen)
Switzerland

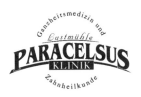

28

Chronic Hypoglycemia, a Common, often Unrecognised, Metabolic Disorder

Introduction

- Does your child suffer from attention disorders, above all before meals? Is he/she often spiteful and bad-tempered and does the teacher complain that his/her performance is very inconsistent?
- Is your child's build rather 'podgy', lacking in tone or even hypotonic?
- Do you as an adult experience tremendous cravings for food and sometimes absolutely have to eat?
- Are you someone who puts on weight even when you really eat very little?
- Do you have a tendency towards obesity or else sometimes unexplained feelings of weakness?
- Do you like carbohydrates such as pasta, potatoes, sweet foods a lot, even though you often feel tired after eating them?
- Do you tend to have feelings of weakness, lose consciousness or feel dizzy?
- Does fasting suit you but only after a few days?
- Does your heart race or does everything go dark sometimes?
- Do you suffer from nervousness, irritability, shivering and anxiety?
- Do you tend to have low blood pressure and rather low body temperatures?

These are questions we ask our patients. If they answer affirmatively, we consider whether they might have a tendency to hypoglycemia or constitutional hyperinsulinemia! It is usually easy to diagnose and also to treat, even though the tendency to hyperinsulinemic hypoglycemia can be only partially modified.

Whilst high blood pressure and diabetes mellitus are extremely well known and also always looked for, chronic hypoglycemia is an almost totally unknown disease even though it is almost as common and can cause the patient severe metabolic problems in the long term, which are often only apparent in poor or inconsistent mental performance but can severely inhibit the sufferer. A tendency to hypoglycemia is usually present from childhood. However with advancing age patients who were previously hypoglycemic often suffer diabetes in old age, as if the decades of excessive insulin production have turned into a weakness of the islet cell system.

Simple biochemistry: human cells need glucose to obtain energy. This is created in the intestine through the splitting of the higher molecule carbohydrates, polysaccharide and disaccharide, into monosaccharides. These are then absorbed from the small intestine and leached into the blood. The subsequent utilization of the sugar (glucose) in the cells is a process dependent on the pancreatic hormone insulin. The more insulin there is present, the faster the sugar seeps into the cells and the blood glucose level drops.

The cell itself does not process the sugar sufficiently fast for the large quantity absorbed and therefore starts an alternative metabolic process of glucose utilization – lipogenesis. In addition, inside the cell the sugar is broken down by fermentation, which leads to local acid production and "over-acidification".

The hypoglycemic patient with an excessive insulin response therefore almost always has raised lipogenesis, in other words fat formation. Their skin symptoms however derive from the excessively low blood sugar levels which arise one or more hours after the intake of food (Figure 1).

Two other possible causes of hypoglycemic metabolic disorder may lie in increased adrenal activity, when the body (adrenal cortex) produces excessive cortisol. There too the raised insulin level is often to be seen as the response.

However the main causes of hypoglycemia are
- First of all malnutrition
- Secondly increased permeability of the intestine
- Thirdly a trace element deficiency

1. Malnutrition

Short chain carbohydrates, such as sugar and sweet foods, but also for example white rice or flour products, are absorbed in the upper tract of the small intestine, sometimes even in the stomach, and are quickly deposited in the blood, so that excessive insulin production occurs, controlled by the hypothalamus. The result is a secondary drop in the blood sugar level (Figure 1).

If the sugar level in the blood drops too low, adrenalin and gluco-corticoids are formed as a compensation mechanism, which charge the liver and release stored carbohydrate (glycogen). The circle is thus closed and even more insulin is produced!

Nutrition tips for hypoglycemic patients:
- No sugar and no foods containing sugar
- No sweet drinks
- Only the smallest quantities of alcohol allowed
- Avoid coffee (adrenal-like effect)
- Very few white flour products

The following are important:
- Plenty of fresh vegetables, raw food, vegetable sprouts and shoots
- Seeds, nuts
- Whole grains such as oats, porridge, spelt, barley etc.
- Raw vegetables as snacks between meals (carrots, organic fennel, avocado etc.)
- Alkaline soup to drink during the day
- Salads with good vegetable oils (olive oil, grapeseed oil, sunflower oil etc.)
- Fruits in the form of non-sulphur-treated dried fruit, as snacks
- Eggs allowed / meat very sparingly / fish once or twice a week

All these foods maintain the blood sugar balance and avoid heavy insulin surges.

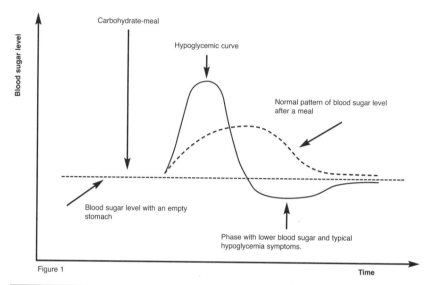

Figure 1

THE PARACELSUS ALKALINE SOUP ACCORDING TO DR. THOMAS RAU

Dr. Rau's alkaline soup is a strongly alkaline-loaded soup, very rich in minerals and particularly suitable for the start of a alkaline diet or fast by Dr. Rau's method, in conjunction with the correction of dietary faults and the accompanying measures in any restorative cure. It provides the body with a surfeit of alkaline foods, and with raw egg yolk added it also supplies high grade fat components, which the body requires for hormone synthesis, among other things adrenalin synthesis, which is very important in exhaustion and in convalescence. This is why this soup, when 3-5 dl are taken every morning, produces an extraordinary stimulating effect, de-acidifies and helps to improve the circadian rhythm, which is often severely disrupted in conditions of adrenal exhaustion.

Preparation: (finely chop the vegetables)
- Celeriac/celery
- Green beans, fresh or frozen, not canned because of the preservatives and sugar
- Courgettes. Always chop this vegetable evenly and moderately finely, in plentiful quantities, so that it "leaches out" well in the decoction
- Instead of beans you can also use lentils, which gives it more protein, or one can add potatoes. Do not add any other vegetables!

Prepare a decoction, leave it to simmer for about 15-20 minutes. Then strain off the vegetables, which might otherwise acidify or ferment.

If necessary you can add some Nahrin stock (vegetable).

No meat stock, no salt.

You can add a raw egg yolk to this bland but very nutritious decoction but only when the mixture is at about 30-50 degrees, so as not to denature the valuable components of the egg yolk. (One egg yolk per person or per large soup bowl). For the purposes of a hypoallergenic diet, do not use hens eggs but quails eggs.

The soup should be eaten the same day and no later than the next day. Try it, you will be amazed at its revitalizing power. It is best not to drink any coffee if you take the soup in the morning. Please note that if you are not eating the soup in conjunction with a fast, you can also eat a small quantity of the vegetables in the evening after you have prepared them, for your evening meal.

2. Permeability of the intestine ("leaky gut syndrome")

The increased permeability of the intestine is due to chemical damage to the mucous membrane of the intestine where there is the wrong intestinal flora or too many preserved foods are being consumed. Another very common cause is food allergy, most commonly an allergy to dairy products. This leads to atrophy of the intestinal mucous membrane and hence its permeability.

For diagnosis thermoregulation diagnostic methods and Vega testing are used to find food allergies, more recently also IgC tests for foods (from Ortho-Analytik).

It is easy to build up the intestinal mucous membrane using Sanum and Burgerstein remedies:

- Notakehl tablets 3x1 for one week
- Then Fortakehl tablets for two weeks
- Then one Mucokehl tablet in the morning and one Nigersan tablet in the evening for several months
- Throughout the whole period Recarcin 6X capsules and Utilin 6X capsules, one of each per week
- One tablet of Burgerstein Molybdenum per day

Dietary:

- Rice gruel daily, no wheat products and no dairy products
- Finely grated raw food, well chewed (cellulose builds up the intestinal bacteria)

A well-known but rarer form of postprandial (= occurring after meals) hypoglycemia is the so-called dumping syndrome in people who have undergone stomach surgery, where the carbohydrates from the meal reach the small intestine and are absorbed there too quickly because of gastric malfunction. This phenomenon can be remedied with small meals, avoidance of sugar and pasta and drinking large quantities of water.

3. Trace element deficiency
The breaking down of glucose requires chromium, manganese, zinc and magnesium. In order to be able to convert glucose to glycogens, in other words to build up stores of carbohydrates, the body requires phosphate, potassium and calcium. Glutamine is important as an amino acid. High levels of copper are counter-productive.

The following regime has proven very beneficial in the treatment of trace element deficiency in hypoglycemia:
- 2 x 10mg manganese
- 2 x 15mg zinc
- 2 x daily glucose tolerance factor (organically bound chromium)
- Also a multivitamin formula such as e.g. the CELA multivitamin and mineral supplement from Burgerstein, 2 x1 tablet daily
- Alkaline remedy recommended: e.g. Burgerstein alkaline mix, 2 x ½ teaspoon per day

Diagnosis of food-related hypoglycemia

1. Hair mineral analysis
On the one hand this reveals any deficiency in hard-to-absorb trace elements: zinc, above all manganese and often also molybdenum. Low chromium is almost pathognomonic in the diagnosis of hypoglycemia! On the other hand the excess acidification which is always present in hypoglycemia leads to calcium and potassium leaking out of the depot, which raises the levels of calcium and magnesium in the Hair Mineral Analysis.

2. Blood sugar and insulin testing after ingestion of glucose (50g glucose in 200ml water)
1-3 hours after taking glucose, the blood sugar level is too low, the insulin

levels are often too high and remain so even when the blood sugar level is once again low.

3. Major stool check orthoanalysis

This reveals miscolonization and also very frequently a reduction in the normal intestinal flora Bifidus and Bacteroides, but also signs of atrophy of the small intestine.

4. Special serum tests

Zinc usually low, vitamin B6 also tends to be low. Histamine values only raised in food allergies. A low spermine level in the serum is also believed to be fairly typical – when it can even be tested in the laboratory.

Summary

- Hypoglycemia is usually food-related and can generally be improved with a consistent change in eating habits!
- Hypoglycemia is very common and usually associated with neurological, metabolic and psychological symptoms.
- Where there is clinical suspicion of hypoglycemia, change of diet, zinc, vitamin B complex, manganese and chromium supplements constitute a very beneficial treatment and produce a clear improvement after about 6-8 weeks.

Dr. Thomas Rau, M.D.
Paracelsus Klinik Lustmühle,
9062 Lustmühle (bei St.Gallen)
Switzerland

Published in Sanum Post No. 60 2002

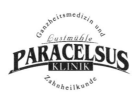

29

Prostate Carcinoma
A Short Review of Biological Cancer Therapy

Prostate cancer is one of the most common illnesses in older men. It is detected in routine examination of the prostate in 20% of the cases in 60 year olds, and in 60% in 80 year olds, even when the patient has had not the slightest complaint or indication. The minor symptoms of prostate cancer in no way represent the seriousness of the disease. A small carcinoma lying in the urethra can, in the earliest phase, get into the blood stream via the sperm or urine. These small carcinomas generally cannot be found this early except through a PSA test, described below.

Lying within the prostate, the cancer tissue frequently cannot be detected for a long time, and causes no discomfort. The typical prostate complaints of slight/reduced urination, occasional burning during urination or difficult urination, or post urination drip are non-specific symptoms which can appear in normal cases as well as in older men experiencing prostate enlargement.

One of the best test options is palpation of the prostate with the finger by a physician able to discover a lump/hardening in the normally elastic prostate tissue. Another very informative early detection test, which also can be part of an appropriate course of treatment, is the test for PSA (Prostate Specific Antigen) in the blood. PSA is a substance that the prostate cancer cells give off, and which can be measured in the blood. As the carcinoma spreads and with the cell growth, PSA values rise, rising particularly with metastasis.

With normal prostate enlargement associated with age and hormonal change, test readings are negative or slightly (to 4.5) raised. With a new test, the PSA can be divided into total and "free" PSA. According to the proportion of plain free flowing PSA relative to the total PSA, normal or abnormal prostate enlargement can be indicated. Another even newer test which is used in the Paracelsus Klinik for early detection of tumor growth is the TPS (Tissue Polypeptide Specific Antigen) test. It indicates early metastasis and tumor growth.

As metastasis appears in the cells, so it frequently spreads to the bones and lymphatic system. Its presence in the bone can be detected via measurement of the alkaline phosphatase in the blood. The more active the bone displacement by cancer cells, the higher the alkaline phosphatase. Somewhat more specific is the so-called Acid Prostate-Phosphatase test. Two other somewhat more costly tests for metastasis are x-ray and Skeletocintigraphy. With this latter test, a small amount of radioactive material is injected and accumulates in the prostate metastasized tissue in the bone, and via a fluororadiography is detected.

Other diagnostic methods for determining cancer tendency, thus early indicators, are the ThermoRegulation Diagnostic, Darkfield Microscopy of the blood, and BioTerrain Assessment. These give indications as to how the carcinoma tendency should be treated and how/which biological therapies should be assembled.

Reflections/Considerations on the Development of Cancer

In the view of holistic medicine, the body must have a tendency towards degeneration, and towards cancer, as a prerequisite for the development of tumors. This tendency towards cancer is often precipitated by the presence of heavy metals in the body, poisons from dental treatments of root canals, trace element deficiencies, extended electro-magnetic loading, also severe emotional stress, vitamin deficiency, etc. The important response is an intensive treatment addressing the degenerative/cancer tendency in addition to the actual tumor treatment. Treatment therapies include vitamin therapy, enzyme therapy, strengthening the immune system, blood cleansing with isopathic therapies, and especially dental assessment with heavy metal removals, the latter being particularly effective against cancer development.

In certain prostate carcinomas, we generally can develop an effective biological approach with a low dose hormone therapy by injection at and around the tumor, within a month bringing down the PSA value.

The physicians at the Paracelsus Klinik in Europe have developed a unique injection therapy in which one is injected at the tumor site with an individual hormone dosage combined with antibody-binding Haptens (specific polysaccharide molecule) and Cytokines (substances which stimulate tumor-killing lymphocytes). Generally with this method, the PSA clearly can be dropped, and particularly when local hyperthermia is employed simultaneously. The drop in PSA indicates a reduction in tumor infiltration and of the tumor itself. This prostate treatment, however, takes some time to effect, at least a year. The results of this treatment are outstanding: According to our observations, 80% of the cases achieve a retreat or, in advanced cases, a stop can be effected.

We do not recommend chemotherapy for prostate carcinoma, as the success rate is very low. Similarly, we seldom recommend surgery early on, as it in most cases offers no more success than other treatments.

Three further important components of prostate cancer treatment are:

1. Local Hyperthermia (Indiba): A heat (interferenzstrom) therapy using current technology with deep heating of the local tissue area; a very high local heating is produced, particularly in firm tissue. Tumor cells do not support/survive this level of heat above 40–44 degrees C. and die back, while healthy tissue is strengthened in the heat; with this treatment, also, metabolism is increased. Thus, the important vital balance can be recovered and surrounding cells improved. This treatment is applied locally and is totally painless. Application is ideally two to three times per week; for some individuals, this treatment works well with fewer applications. This therapy is a specialty of the Paracelsus Klinikg and is practiced nowhere else in Switzerland. Within about twenty treatments, the tumor tissue can be regenerated bringing about a scarring over and connective tissue change in the tumor.

2. Mistletoe Therapy: Mistletoe therapy with an injection of a mistletoe preparation is the best studied/researched tumor treatment, and at Paracelsus the pillar of tumor treatments. We employ the injection preparation Iscador from the firm Weleda; it is the best-made and most effective preparation, composed of mistletoe plants grown on pines or oaks (Iscador Qu). The preparations are injected subcutaneously in the groin/abdomen by the patient in increasing dosages twice weekly. The patient is taught the simple injection technique.

3. The above mentioned local **"Neuraltherapy"** injection: The tumor is injected with a very specific preparation of low dose natural hormone, isopathic and homeopathic medications in a special base mix, causing reduced growth and reduction of the malignancy in the tumor cells.

4. In addition to the specifically named cancer treatments we follow an on-going protocol of rebuiding and **strengthening the inner milieu and immune system;** of treatment and removal/elimination of all factors which lead to the malignant degeneration of the tissue. We call these therapies the holistic "basic cancer treatment." They include the administration of trace elements, minerals, isopathic medications according to Prof. Enderlein, enzymes, haptens, etc. An important part of the treatment is the rehabilitation from toxic loading of such heavy metals like mercury, etc., which stressed the immune system, as well as toxins from dental treatment of root canals.

Dr. Thomas Rau, M.D.
Paracelsus Klinik Lustmühle,
9062 Lustmühle (bei St.Gallen)
Switzerland

Paracelsus information leaflet 2001
Copyright © 2001 Dr. Thomas Rau
All Rights Reserved

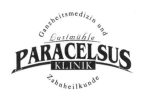

30

Dr. Rau's comments and explanations on Brain Tumours

GLIOBLASTOMA in adults is normally a very malignant brain tumour, which develops very fast and leads to neurological problems by compression of the normal brain tissue and also by infiltration of the nerval tissue or the stem ganglia. The consequences therefore are high pressure of the brain fluid and also cerebral paralysis.

Orthodox medicine treats this kind of tumour with surgery, chemotherapy and radiation. The options are limited by the site of the tumour. The deeper the tumour and the closer it is to the stem ganglia, the more difficult it gets to treat. Radiation also damages the brain tissue and is therefore very problematic. Different types of chemo therapy are administered, but also have a limited effect.

The prognosis of this tumour is very bad. Over 50% of patients die within two years after diagnosis. The 5 year survival rate is below 10%, if treated by allopathic medicine.

Therefore treatment has to be either supplemented by or totally carried out by Integrated Biological Medicine, which addresses to the causes of the disease such as toxins, free radicals, decreased immune system and electromagnetic or geopathic load. Most patients have high **heavy metal levels** which suppress the immune system and disturb the glia cells so much that they can develop into cancerous cells. (Histochemical analyses of Glioblastoma tissue have shown highly elevated levels of mercury concentration.)

There is a Indian plant remedy which we use and has shown amazing effects arresting or decelerating the course of the glioblastoma disease up to 60%. 30% of cases were significantly arrested! The name of the drug is **Boswellia Serrata** (incente from special Indian incense-trees). This substance has to be given in a very pure, high dosage for at least 6 months.

Very frequently we also find **neurotropic viruses,** which can also cause glioblastoma. Neurotrophic viruses are viruses which normally do not trigger cerebral disease, but in the course of a longterm infection then can produce longterm brain cell irritation, which then leads to cancer. These viruses (for example Herpes, FSME, LCM-virus) are found in the blood by elevated antiviral antibodies. Treatment is done by homeopathic nosodes and catalysts.

Our experiences using this combined treatment are quite good, compared to orthodox medicine: patients normally feel better, the course of the disease is slowed down or stopped. Many patients have much less side-effects from allopathic medicine methods, such as chemotherapy and radiation.

The methods we use are: detoxification, mercury removal, elimination of disturbances foci (teeth, tonsils, etc.), immune-stimulating i.v.'s and cytokines and haptenes, isopathic remedies according to Prof. Enderlin and high dosages of vitamins, according to individual tests and redox potential analysis (BTA).

In addition to Boswellia Serrata given in high dosages, another specialized treatment at the Paracelsus Clinic is local hyperthermia, a deep interference electron-transmittant hyperthermia, given locally to the tumour site, which does not hurt the surrounding tissue. Such a treatment cure lasts about 3–4 weeks. Mistletoe Injections and special hapten (tumour-antigens) injections are added to the program.

Dr. Thomas Rau, M.D.
Paracelsus Klinik Lustmühle,
9062 Lustmühle (bei St.Gallen)
Switzerland

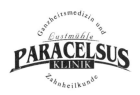

31

Options in the Biological Therapy of Hypertension

From a holistic medicinal viewpoint, hypertension is a classical regulation phenomenon, in which the body attempts to increase circulation – especially microcirculation – by elevating blood pressure, so that oxygen supply to the tissues will improve. This has usually deteriorated because the patient has reduced oxygenation and deoxygenation erythrocyte function, or because the interstitial tissue has become less oxygen-permeable.

Inspecting the blood under the dark-field, one sees extensive rouleau formation and, frequently, thick protein borders all around the erythrocytes. According to Prof. Enderlein's isopathic teachings, hypertension patients usually exhibit massive amounts of endobiontic valences.

Therefore, hypertension must be treated along the following lines:

- **Milieu change**

The interstitial spaces substance transport capability must be improved: deacidification and deproteinization with dietary readjustment, trace elements, alkaline therapy:

Multivitamins: Cela Burgerstein, 2 per day.

ALKALA: $^1/_2$ to 1 measuring spoon per day, taken in hot water; in the morning, a diet low in animal protein and milk-free.

(Milk protein is reabsorbed well from the intestines, but increases viscosity in the interstitium (congestion). This then reduces substance – and thus also oxygen – transport to the cells. Therefore, any hyperprotein condition leads to "under nutrition" and premature cell aging.)

- **Isopathic Therapy of Hypertension**
  (combined with milieu therapy):
  Must be long-term (at least 1 year).
  Mucor racemosus 5X tablets: 2 in the morning, 1 at noon; after one month, cut back to 1 tablet each morning and noon.
  SANUVIS drops: 40 drops thrice daily (duration of therapy: a few months).
  Dextrorotary lactic acid (Homaccord) improves cell respiration.

- **Homeopathic treatment**
  Must be done on an individual basis. Often there is a good response to Rauwolfia preparations, Solidago preparations and compound agents such as Co-Hypert (Pekana).

- **Improvement of cell respiration**
  Reduced cell respiration and oxygen exchange puts the tissue cells into a deficiency condition. Therefore, cellular metabolism must be improved. This is accomplished by means of the above-named Cela vitamin preparations, but also with coenzvmes such as Coenzvme comp. (Heel), one ampule thrice weekly; subcutaneously or orally. Alternative: catalysts from the citric acid cycle (10 ampules per package, 10 different enzymes/ catalysts of the citric acid cycle, take an ampule combined every other day.

  Very important: focus cleansing. Impacted wisdom teeth (heart/small intestine meridian) and root-canaled front teeth (kidney/bladder meridian) are especially bad. These must always be cleansed.

Dr. Thomas Rau, M.D.
Paracelsus Klinik Lustmühle,
9062 Lustmühle (bei St.Gallen)
Switzerland

Translated and published by Explore! Volume 8, Number 1, 1997

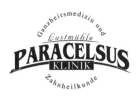

32

The risks of immunisation against hepatitis B
The problems from a holistic point of view

Preliminary remarks by the Editor:
For many years it was compulsory in Germany for children to be immunised against smallpox. If parents omitted to have their children immunised they could be punished. There were not many qualified people who warned against smallpox immunisation and even in the early days forecast that this mass immunisation would result in some children becoming dangerously ill. But the warnings were deliberately ignored and thrown to the winds, the authorities continuing to threaten parents who looked into the matter in a deeper and responsible manner with penalties if they did not have their children immunised. The fact that the compulsory requirement for immunisation was in fact finally lifted after a period of hesitation which was all too long, does corroborate – albeit belatedly – the views of the people who had been giving the warnings, but the damage caused by immunisation is serious and in a significant number of cases cannot be reversed. What is now threatening people affected by the promotion of hepatitis inoculations, because the earlier damage has been disregarded? The following contribution by Dr Thomas Rau MD tries to throw light on this problem. The enormous complexity and seriousness of the problem of inoculation in general has already been addressed in the article "Inoculations and the consequences of inoculation" by Dr Thomas Rau MD in SANUM Post 46 beginning on page 15.

Older schoolchildren in Switzerland are sent an official letter of information recommending that they should have themselves immunised against hepatitis B. This calls for closer investigation of a problem which unfortunately is being disregarded in this instance but can be seen when one looks at the matter from a holistic viewpoint. From this point of view, the recommendation of immunisation provokes great scepticism and doubt.

Immunisation programmes of this type have already been carried out in France, the USA and other countries. Because of serious criticism and doubt on the part of practitioners of holistic medicine, but also among the population as a whole, in France these immunisation programmes have already been suspended and in one instance in the USA the compulsory requirement for immunisation has been lifted. This shows that the enormous doubts that have been expressed are justified.

In the case of the hepatitis B vaccine in common use, immunisation is carried out using a living virus which is produced from living cell cultures and has been altered by means of genetic manipulation. It is already a matter for alarm that it is not yet possible to foresee the long-term effects of this gene manipulation, as techniques of vaccine production like this have only been in use for about 10 years. As a general rule, the problematic long-term effects of vaccines can only be assessed after 15 to 20 years.

The cell cultures used for the production of vaccine are animal cell cultures of which the purity and safety cannot be guaranteed with any certainty. In other countries it has already been suggested that other viruses which cannot yet be identified are also being passed on through the hepatitis vaccines. The discussion on this subject in the USA is revealing: some people regard the spread of HIV (the AIDS virus) as being connected with the use of this vaccine and other live virus vaccines. In any case, it is known that other vaccines can lead to sensitisation of the carrier cells, causing an allergy to protein. This can result in many allergies to animals with accompanying skin problems, asthma, etc., like that already known in immunisation against diphtheria and whooping cough.

Every inoculation using a live virus leads to an infection with altered viruses which for the most part only cause underlying clinical characteristics of the disease, but in fact have an effect which is so strong that as a result a virus whose long-term effect is still unknown can cause a chronic infection. This justifies the considerable reservations. It has already been possible to establish that in the case of other vaccines produced by similar methods for immunisation against measles, polio and mumps, long-term infections which give cause for alarm have arisen with increasing frequency at a later date. These often appeared only after a period of several years, mainly in the form of chronic allergic diseases, chronic brain problems and disorders of the central nervous system. But we still know too little about these risks in order to be able to exclude them with any accuracy.

To be sure, the hepatitis virus can represent a potential danger in people with a weak immune system and in the corresponding accompanying illnesses. However in most cases the infection is not expressed as a tangible illness but is "processed" by the immune system of the infected person. In any case, the risk of a young person suffering a severe attack of hepatitis B or C is relatively small. In biological treatment which is professional, i.e. builds the patient up, the virus infection can in most cases be completely cured without later effects. Against this backdrop one gets the impression that the promotion of immunisation against hepatitis is upheld by a fear which can hardly be properly justified.

The hepatitis B virus is transferred in the same way as the AIDS virus. Therefore it is urgently recommended that one should take the same protective measures as against AIDS, including during sexual contact, in order to protect oneself equally against hepatitis B and also hepatitis C. At the same time it must be considered that the hepatitis B immunisation being recommended does not "protect" against hepatitis C, hepatitis A or the hepatitis connected with mononucleosis. People who have been immunised should therefore not make false assumptions that they are safe.

One problem which has not yet been explained or refuted occurred in the Paris region, where about 450'000 children and adolescents were immunised: it was reported that within two years 578 cases of MS-type illness had occurred in those people who had been immunised. That is about eighty times more than the usual occurrence of MS illnesses in the population. These complications led to immunisation against hepatitis B in the Paris region being halted. To be sure, no corresponding study on the subject has yet been completed, nor is there yet any final definite certainty in the way the problem is being refuted, but in view of this development it could clearly be too early to carry out immunisation programmes with the same hepatitis B vaccine in Switzerland or elsewhere.

From the point of view of the doctor's responsibility, we should therefore be advising against the immunisation of healthy children and young people. There is the danger of consequential damage, even if cannot be fully understood at the present time. the risk following immunisation cannot be justifiably compared with the much smaller risk of actually becoming ill with hepatitis. The anti-viral immunity of young people can be strengthened quite substantially by biological means using other methods including isopathic remedies, and in this way a good level of protection is also given against other viral illnesses.

Dr. Thomas Rau, M.D.
Paracelsus Klinik Lustmühle,
9062 Lustmühle (bei St.Gallen)
Switzerland

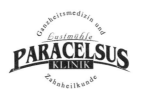

33

On the Value of Darkfield Microscopy: Corroboration of Diagnosis with Live Blood in a Variety of Cases

The Paracelsus Klinik in Switzerland is a well-known clinic which successfully uses many tried and tested therapeutic procedures of Integrated Biological Medicine under the direction of experienced doctors with comprehensive university qualifications. In this clinic the most important of the tried and tested tools is darkfield microscopy using the patient's live blood. It has proved itself over a number of years as a reliable and essential means of establishing a diagnosis and is an integral part of the doctor's assessment of the patient's regulatory ability. In this way of looking at Integrated Biological Medicine, illness is not regarded as a phenomenon of an isolated disorder of an organ but as a disorder of a dynamic process of regulation which involves the whole organism.

That is why whole-body metabolic processes, the regulatory processes of the homeostasis and the whole organism's ability to adapt are the deciding factors for a person's health. And it is these functions and abilities in particular which can be assessed very successfully with the aid of darkfield microscopic investigation of live blood. This also applies particularly to control and documentation of the desirable progress in a complete course of therapy.

Darkfield microscopy – its use and evidence
In darkfield investigations a drop of fresh blood is examined under the microscope without staining. The blood taken from the patient is thus put directly onto the slide and covered with a glass cover slip. The slide is

examined immediately under 1200x magnification. The blood is then exposed to severe stress in the slide preparation through lack of oxygen, non-circulation and exposure to light. After the blood has been subjected to this stress, the image which appears under the microscope allows important conclusions to be drawn about the resistance of the cells to changes in redox and oxygen and, like time-lapse photography, it can display the rate of tendency of the blood and its cells to degenerate better than any other test. The insights offered by the microscopic image include among other things the significant signs of change in the important acid-base balance and thus the milieu for the development of microbes and the resistance of the cell walls.

Darkfield microscopy also offers insights of particular interest into the protein content of cells, the activities of leucocytes and the tendency to degenerate up to the point where a malignancy threatens or starts. In this way – assuming appropriate experience on the part of the investigator – this method of investigation enables many conclusions to be drawn about the dynamic processes and sequence of events in the organism of the patient. This very dynamic is an important characteristic for a reliable assessment of the patient, whilst on the other hand the ways of looking at it which in many cases are statistical and only concerned with the organs miss the living reality.

Darkfield microscopy therefore does not offer a specific organ diagnosis or a nosological diagnosis; instead its core evidence is concerned with stresses which cause illness and tendencies to disease, as found primarily in the circulatory system. The conclusions resulting from the live blood in the darkfield, as regards the ability to function and the cell resistance of the leucocytes, are of particular value for clarifications in the area of immune disorders and tumours. This applies above all to the question of tolerability of immune-suppressive and chemotherapy drugs. Darkfield microscopy therefore also offers benefits for its use in conventional oncology.

The research carried out by Professor Enderlein is definitely the basis of all darkfield microscope investigations carried out in the clinic, but the more recent findings and experiences of many competent investigators have also become part of this method. Whilst in Germany many hundreds of practices regularly use darkfield microscopy for the assessment of the condition of their patients' illnesses, in the USA there are already more than one thousand doctors who use it to form their diagnosis. This tendency is increasing and the level of interest is continuing to grow, so that the regular courses which began years ago for doctors and non-medical practitioners to learn about darkfield microscopy continue to be held. The organiser of these courses for beginners and advanced practitioners is the International Society for Milieu Therapy, Isopathy and Darkfield Microscopy for doctors and natural health practitioners in Lustmühle, Switzerland.

An overall view of the possibilities of darkfield microscopy

To put it briefly, darkfield microscopic investigation of the living blood gives early reliable insights into tendencies towards illness of different kinds, including tendencies towards circulatory, dysbiotic and degenerative malign illnesses. For this the following signs in particular should be looked for in the microscopic picture:

- Shifts in the acid-base metabolism

- Shortcomings in the digestion of proteins because of an image of "rouleau" in the blood, of changes in the redox potential and precipitation of fibrin in the blood

- Tendency for cells to degenerate

- Anisocytosis, chronic inflammations and disorders of absorption of iron

- Accelerated atrophy of the cells

- Autolysis of the leukocytes caused by contamination by toxins

- Cellular endobiontic contamination

- Upward development of endobiontic high valencies which cause illness

- Dysbiosis

  and
- Assessment of the "blood milieu"

The last-named symptom is revealed in the microscopic image in the course of further darkfield investigation by the fast development of bacterial valencies. This picture is found in many patients and enables illnesses which may become serious later to be effectively treated in this early stage by methods which do not allow them to reach the serious stage. This benefit of early assessment using darkfield microscopy must again be stressed, as this method enables a course of treatment to be undertaken which can result in real and complete healing of the condition.

Dr. Thomas Rau, M.D.
Paracelsus Klinik Lustmühle,
9062 Lustmühle (bei St.Gallen)
Switzerland

Published in Sanum Post No. 50 2000

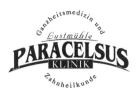

34

The isopathic principle

Testing medicines using a darkfield microscope

In this paper Dr. Rau once again explains the possibility of checking the effect of isopathic medicines using a darkfield microscopic image of vital blood. This method of testing has already been used by Professor Enderlein as an important instrument in developing the SANUM products.

In darkfield microscopy, if, a few minutes to one hour after taking a blood sample, one drop of an isopathic medicine is carefully added to the prepared sample, a massive reduction in the high and medium valencies can be observed, provided the right isopathic SANUM medicine has been chosen.

The following different phenomena are frequently observed:

- cells "lose" their luminous, thick cell walls, individual cells turn into "shadow cells" with just the thinnest of cell walls remaining, as thecites the size of erythrocytes.

  It is thought that this is because the endobiontic middle valencies on the cell walls are reduced by the chondrites or spermites of the isopathic products, causing a copulative valency reduction.

- High valencies such as chondrites, bacteria phases or even ascites are broken down and a very large number of low valencies occurs e.g. macrosymprotites.

- If one then simply leaves the sample to stand, over the course of several hours, or up to one day, high valencies develop again, but in a great variety and many forms, often as bizarre high valency images, with very many different high to low valencies. This is an image which otherwise, without the administration of isopathic agents, one sees only occasionally in highly reactive patients, after long-lasting SANUM therapy or in children with inflammatory conditions.

- In my view and on the basis of Enderlein's explanation, these two phenomena are the expression of the great endobiontic regulatory effectiveness of the deep valencies contained in the isopathic agent. They are therefore quite rightly called "regulators".

First of all they diminish the high valencies through reduction or copulation and form a gigantic number of the lowest valencies, in other words a plethoric situation, which one would have to eliminate from a living patient and maintain them at low valency with alkali and mineral therapy. That is why it is so very important for the isopathy to be accompanied by orthomolecular and alkaline therapy!

In the darkfield preparation this accompanying environmental therapy naturally does not take place, so that the endobiontic low valencies formed increase again in the pathological, anaerobic and over-alkaline, haemolytic environmental situation of the prepared sample. However if they do not encounter any blockades, they also develop in an extremely wide variety of forms.

The darkfield test with isopathic remedies is a very valuable test to check how far the patient's blood can be regulated and how much the environment can change. It can also provide indications of other regulatory blockades such as dental focus toxins or heavy metals, since there too there are no different high valencies developed, but a strikingly high number of mono-forms such as, for example, typically mychites (bacteria phases) in the presence of root toxins (teeth with root fillings and mesenchymal toxin leaching).

Dr. Thomas Rau, M.D.
Paracelsus Klinik Lustmühle,
9062 Lustmühle (bei St.Gallen)
Switzerland

Published in SANUM Post No. 48 1999

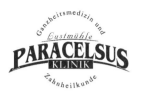

35

Evaluation of Hair Mineral Analysis and its Significance for Isopathic and Regulation Medicine

INTRODUCTION AND GENERAL CONSIDERATIONS

Regulation and Mineral Salts

Regulation means recognizing changing environmental conditions and adapting to them. The goal of regulation is to establish internal equilibrium at the cellular, tissue and organism levels. But the cell's regulatory and reactive ability depends considerably on the its ability to maintain its internal equilibrium, i.e. maintain a redox and membrane potential of ca. 60-80 mV (as opposed to a reduced potential in degenerate or cancerous cells of ca. 40-60 mV).

This depends, in turn, on the exchange of electrolytes and trace elements through the cell wall, as well as on the presence of catalysts for chemical cellular processes. Thus, the presence of electrolytes and trace elements is immensely important for the cell's reactive ability. Therefore, when the cellular (but also interstitial) mineral salts, electrolytes, trace elements change, no regulative therapy can function properly.

An orthomolecular assessment (and treatment) of the patient is thus a prerequisite for any regulative therapy. The Sanum firm takes this into account in its palette of remedies, by offering mineral salts and vitamins (such as Mapurit or Seleno-methionine), as well as highly potentiated homeopathic agents with catalytic effects on cellular chemical activity such as Pleo Zinc, Pleo Cup, Selenokehl.

Isopathy and Orthomolecular Therapy

Sanum therapeutic agents, particularly the Isopathic remedies, are medications which influence regulatory ability, either by altering the cellular organelles and thus cellular chemical activity, or by modifying the interstitial fluids. Therefore, recognizing and dealing with changing environmental conditions is closely tied to isopathic as well as to the orthomolecular relationship. Isopathy and orthomolecular therapy are thus closely allied and complement each other marvellously, as has been confirmed many times over in the context of the acid-base balance. So it is understandable that we, as holistic physicians, should look for ways to assess the orthomolecular relationships.

Methods for Assessing the Orthomolecular and Milieu Relationships

Acid-Base Balance
    Urine tests
Blood Tests
    Redox potential
    Mineral salts
    Trace elements
Hair Mineral Analyses

Hair Mineral Analysis

Assessing the mineral salt content (plus heavy metals and other toxic substances) in the organism is thus often very important for the biologically-oriented physician, in order to be able to evaluate regulatory blockages, but also to be able to recognize the orthomolecular substitution requirements. The problem is that these substances are present in part intracellularly, and thus not significantly in the usual test media such as blood, urine and stool. This is the case for all the mineral salts, whether present intracellularly, at the cells or in the lymphatic regions.

We know, for example, that iron content is very reduced in chronic inflammation cases – not in the organism as a whole, but rather it's shifted into connective-tissue depots and the liver. So it makes no sense to determine serum iron in chronic inflammation cases – and it makes even less sense to institute iron therapy because of a low serum iron level, which could even turn out to be harmful to the mesenchyme. Instead, what is important – from a biological regulative standpoint – is to improve the iron uptake in the cell by administering zinc. So, what is needed is a test that can detect the presence of iron (and zinc) elsewhere, namely intracellularly.

The situation is similar for very many other mineral salts and trace elements, whose content is only significant intracellularly or fixed in cells, such as nearly all the heavy metals, as well as the trace elements necessary to the citric acid cycle, such as zinc, chromium, manganese. For these substances, hair mineral analysis is particularly significant, since it tests the cellular content of these elements.

The Dynamics of Mineral-Salt Uptake

It is very important that the results of Hair Mineral Analysis not be interpreted in a "one-to-one" manner, i.e. not looking at one mineral at a time in isolation, but instead interrelatedly. For example, if there is a deficiency, one should always check for possible high levels of the corresponding antagonist, such as mercury and selenium or aluminum and zinc. For example, if aluminum is high – which is extremely common in Switzerland (and often correlated with neurological problems) – then this is especially relevant when the regular antagonists zinc and/or manganese are low, or (as a sign of a hyperacidic condition) calcium and magnesium or phosphate are high.

The combined "assessment of Hair Mineral Analysis as a unit" is thus important and can say a lot about resorption ability, enteral situation, intestinal permeability, as well as interstitial information transfer, etc. A mineral salt, trace element or toxic substance is introduced, taken up and only then actively resorbed through the intestinal mucous membrane, then "rinsed" through the Peyer's plaques, transported via the lymphatic system (depending on the lymph's transport capacity) and only then taken into the tissue cells. But there are also substances which diffuse across concentration gradients, i.e. are present in higher concentration in cases involving thinner and damaged intestinal mucosa, such as lead and aluminum.

WHAT HAIR MINERAL ANALYSIS SAYS ABOUT THE ENTERAL SITUATION

Active Enteral Resorption

Trace elements, which have to be actively and cellularly resorbed through the mucosa from the intestinal lumen, are reduced in cases involving intestinal mucosal atrophy. Intestinal mucosal atrophy is often brought about by dietary allergies and point to mast-cell degranulation in the intestinal lumen and thus cellular degeneration. Intestinal mucosa which has been damaged to such a degree can no longer properly handle cellular resorption of zinc, resulting in a zinc deficiency in the body (and in the hair). Thus, the zinc deficiency is not a cause, but rather an effect of the dietary allergy. Now, if this zinc deficiency is also found along with an elevated aluminum level, then the likelihood of a dietary allergy is even greater, since, in cases of intestinal mucosal atrophy, aluminum – a typical diffusion element – can diffuse better through the intestinal wall.

Zinc itself, as a cellularly active resorption element, is thereby subject to very many factors:

- Antagonism to cadmium, copper, lead content
- Dietary content of zinc-binding phytic acid
- Calcium content and alkalinity of the intestinal contents
- Parasites and other chronic inflammatory intestinal diseases

But zinc itself also catalytically enables incorporation of iron into hemoglobin, so that, specifically in cases involving chronic inflammatory anemias, the binding of iron should be ensured with zinc, i.e. zinc should also be administered for iron deficiency, so as to improve the anemia and the "iron deficiency".

Manganese and Chromium

The situation is similar for other active cellularly reabsorbed elements. If all of these are low in the Hair Mineral Analysis, this points to cellular mucosal reabsorption disorders. On the other hand, if in addition the "diffusion elements" are elevated, then one may much more confidently conclude that the intestinal mucosa are damaged, i.e. a "leaky gut syndrome" is present and, above all, the intestinal mucosa and the intestinal flora which seal them need to be built up.

The Hair Mineral Analysis therefore yields information not only about mineral-salt requirements and the need for detoxification, but also intestinal flora, intestinal permeability and quality of the mucosa – thus excellently supplementing other regulative medical diagnostic procedures such as darkfield microscopy, Rost's thermoregulation diagnostics and redox potential determination.

In this context, chromium is somewhat of a special case, in that chromium is used in large amounts by the pancreas cells in the production of insulin; thus, when there is a cellular chromium deficiency in the Hair Mineral Analysis, one should consider a cellular chromium deficiency in the pancreas, and in the parotid gland as well – with corresponding diabetic or enzymatic problems.

Passive Enteral Diffusion

All heavy metals and toxic metals which have a negative effect on the immune system, pass out of the intestines via diffusion, and can diffuse to a greater degree if the intestinal mucosa are in poor condition, thus showing up to a greater degree in the Hair Mineral Analysis. Now, if a child with a high susceptibility to infection has low zinc and high aluminum in the Hair Mineral Analysis, possibly also high lead and maybe even low manganese, then therapy should primarily concentrate on the intestines, using isopathic and homeopathic means to build the intestinal flora back up (see below). If, in addition, iron is reduced (actually fairly rare), then an added dysbiotic or pancreatic disorder is almost certainly present. If the little patient then has foul-smelling flatulence (as an expression of disturbed cellulose processing due to pancreatic insufficiency), then we know that we have to concentrate on the intestinal flora and the pancreas, using Sanum products and building up the intestinal flora: Pleo Fort tablets, 1 tablet 3 times daily, Glucose Tolerance Factor, Pleo Reb 4X capsules. So, along with the orthomolecular substitution, the indication for the type of intestinal therapy can also be determined with the Hair Mineral Analysis.

Mesenchymal Transport Routes

As intercellular space, the mesenchyme is interspersed with extremely fine nerve endings, polysaccharide molecules, fibrocytes and interstitial fluid. All nutrients must pass through this interstitial space on the way to the cell. Fine-material/energetic information can only be passed on by means of changes in the interstitial fluid.

As the most important intracorporeal transport and information route, interstitial tissue is very dependent on the interstitial fluid, characterized by its dissolved polysaccharide molecules and their directedness, and water-molecule clustering. It could thus be shown that the composition of the interstitial fluid is largely characterized by the mineral salts and trace elements dissolved in it. Quartz, the epitome of geometric structure, is the element used in information transmission. We know this function of silicon from computer science, where it is used as a basic element in computer chips. But it is also an important mediator of structure in man, for which the prerequisites are combinatorial and informational capabilities. Thus, silicon is the element of the mesenchyme, but also of orientation and support of the individual in the environment. As a trace element, silicon is thus to be categorized with interstitial tissue in Hair Mineral Analysis.

When Hair Mineral Analysis indicates a silicon deficiency, one may assume that the patient will not respond very well to energetic methods, and not only needs to have silicon substitution, but also to undergo mesenchymal treatment with compensation techniques, etc. The situation for the electrolytes sodium and potassium is similar, although they are subject to greater error values in Hair Mineral Analysis.

SPECIAL DISEASE PICTURES IN HAIR MINERAL ANALYSIS

Hyperacidity

Hyperacidity is a very common problem, usually chronic and also usually dietarily conditioned. Detecting it is usually clinically possible, but difficult to confirm in the laboratory. Test methods are mostly confined to fluid media to the exclusion of cells and tissues.

Hair Mineral Analysis offers some indications of hyperacidity:

- **Calcium and magnesium high:** the calcium deposits are being mobilized out of the bones to buffer acid-equivalents (usually unmetabolized amino acid due to excess protein) and to bind them into protein-mineral complexes. Calcium and magnesium are mobilized to a greater degree and thus appear in higher concentrations in the cells and hairs.
- **Phosphorus is often elevated.** Phosphorus has a close relationship with magnesium. Phosphorus deficiency often appears in conjunction with magnesium deficiency, and phosphorus is mobilized out of the bones much as magnesium is. However, it is contained in acidic substances such as meat, sausage products, cheese, dairy products, nuts, chocolate and preserved foods.
- **Aluminum often high:** aluminum's solubility depends directly on the pH of the liquid that it is dissolved in. Nowadays, aluminum is, first, more dissolved in today's more acid-heavy bodily fluids and, second, taken up through the hair. In Switzerland, most aluminum comes from the water supply: for one thing, water is increasingly acidic, plus it also contains increasing quantities of fine suspended matter, representing mostly negatively-charged proteins to which the aluminum cation can be bound.

Aluminum, and lead as well, is bound to a greater degree by the (in our opinion) inadvisable – not to say dangerous – practice of chlorinating drinking water (with aluminum chloride): the negatively-charged chloride binds with the cation $Pb+$ or $Al++$. The situation is similar for suspended protein matter in drinking water, whose negative charge binds to the cations Al, Pb and Hg. Which explains why the main source of aluminum pollution comes from drinking water. This also explains our recommendation to rid drinking water of suspended matter via reflux osmosis. Aluminum is also important for other disease pictures which also happen to involve hyperacidity.

The Hyperactive Child

An investigation by the child psychologist Dr. W. Egli (Ennetbaden, Switzerland) has shown – a very interesting connection – a close correlation between hyperactivity and high aluminum levels in the Hair Mineral Analysis.

Our view is that a child's hyperactive syndrome is a classical poly-causal functional disorder, on the one hand often having toxic components, but on the other also abnormal intestinal bacterial flora and/or dietary allergies as causes. We thus usually observe similar shifts in the Hair Mineral Analysis of children with heightened susceptibility to disease and those with dietary allergies. Therefore, we always treat the hypermotoric child with isopathic agents as well (see therapy plan below).

Another finding: one often sees reduced manganese in the Hair Mineral Analyses of hyperactive children. Manganese is a very important intracellular catalytic trace element, but it is generally quite unknown. As manganophosphoric acid, it is a catalyst in the citric acid cycle, therefore intervening centrally in cellular energy metabolism. This also explains why brain-metabolic symptoms such as hyperactivity appear in deficiency cases.

Similarly, with syndromes like this, the other trace elements involved in cell metabolism, such as iodine, chromium and lithium, are often also reduced. The combination of high toxic metals and low catalyst/trace elements is quite typical of the hyperactive child. Always keep milk-protein allergies (and concomitant hyperacidity) in mind as well.

AN EXAMPLE

Daniel S., 6-Year-Old Child

Main problem: behavioural disorders; hyperactivity, speech problems, fine motor disorders, disease susceptibility, tonsil operation, various antibiotic cures.

It is worth mentioning that the child had already been following a diet based on subtle energetic testing, plus had been taking evening primrose oil, zinc and multivitamins, with no effect on the clinical situation. The clinical examination showed a saliva test value of pH 5.8 and fissured, somewhat macerated anal mucous membrane as signs of dysbiosis. Plus the typical findings of the somewhat retarded leptosomatic child, somewhat fidgety, lightly bulged cutaneous turgor.

The Hair Mineral Analysis was done because, despite the usual orthomolecular catching therapy (see above), no change could be achieved. One expects the Hair Mineral Analysis to bring out additional aspects. Besides the Hair Mineral Analysis, a darkfield vital blood examination was also made to assess the "inner milieu", as well as a "Dry Layer Test" of the blood. The findings of the Hair Mineral Analysis are reproduced below. They show – despite the zinc and vitamin substitution, a general deficiency picture: in the upper section, the mineral salts and trace elements are reduced throughout. (It is worth mentioning that certain substances were even below the detection limits and were thus not even entered into the chart (Mo, Co, V, Ge).

Zinc, chromium and manganese were particularly reduced, despite rather good "hyperacidity parameters" (Ca, Mg, pH). Iodine – metabolic agent – was likewise reduced. With findings like this, it would have been useless to simply supply the deficient substances, as had already been done, because of the certain presence (reasons given below) of a resorption disorder, which in this case can be impressively derived from the Hair Mineral Analysis data.

The therapy will not then be purely orthomolecular, but rather must encompass – with Sanum remedies – rebuilding up the intestinal mucosa and flora.

The assumption of intestinal resorption and mucosa disorders can be made based on the following combination:

- Reduction of nearly all cellular-resorptive trace elements: Zn, Cr, Mn, I, Fe
- Elevated toxic diffusing heavy metals (Al, Pb, Cd)
- Hyperacidity findings very limited

(To which should be added that children, in their already mostly anabolic condition, are usually alkaline and thus seldom exhibit the typical calcium-magnesium shifts.)

A darkfield microscopic examination of vital blood was carried out as a supplementary test; it showed a massive milieu shift as well as excess protein with signs of overburdened leukocytes and lymphocytes – i.e., once again the findings of digestive disorders on the protein level as well, with consequent immune overstress.

The toxic minerals/metals aluminum and lead largely explain the neurological symptomatology, including fidgetiness, retarded development, attention disorders, etc., in that they reduce the stimulus threshold of the nerves. The deficiency of the antagonists Zn, Mn and Cr exarcebates the condition and again reinforces the suspicion of damaged intestinal mucous membranes.

SAMPLE ANALYSIS

Age: 6 Gender: M Name: Daniel

Technically ideal smear
- Cells medium strong endobiontic burden, strong flickering, as for Mucor
- Unclear but very extended mycelium-like fibers
- Dioekothecits in huge numbers, as expression of excessive reactivity
- Liver nicely active
- Protits extremely lively
- Massive milieu changes
- Toxic problems
- Profound milieu disturbances, changed structure of intestinal mucous membrane, excretion of huge amounts of toxins

Isopathy
Therapy was aimed at the milieu and intestinal mucous membrane, as well as the basic cause.

Dietary allergy. The basic dietary allergies, milk and eggs, had to be avoided. In addition, the mucosa and immune system were built up using Sanum remedies:

Pleo Sancom, Pleo Reb capsules, Pleo Ut and Pleo Rec in drops and capsules later.

Sample Analysis

Age: **6**   Gender: **M**   **Daniel**
Test date: 1/31/97   Ref Nr: 23440   Dr. Thomas Rau
Hair Mineral Analyses: values in ppm (parts per million)
Calcium values over 2000 and magnesium values over 200 indicate a deficiency condition, in which the body increasingly mobilizes (i.e. acquires) these elements out of its reserves (solid tissue such as bones).

MINERAL	REFERENCE RANGE	TEST VALUE	LOW	NORMAL	HIGH
Ca (calcium)	450-1550	936			
Mg (magnesium)	30-180	50			
P (phosphorus)	135-275	154			
Zn (zinc)	240-320	220			
Cr (chromium)	0.4-0.6	0.25			
Mn (manganese)	0.3-1.4	0.20			
Mo (molybdenum)	0.1-0.8	<0.11			
Cu (copper)	8-24	15.4			
Fe (iron)	12-24	11.4			
Se (selenium)	0.3-0.9	0.4			
I (iodine)	12-35	8.9			
S (sulfur)	31,000-47,000	44,645			
Na (sodium)	40-130	15			
K (potassium)	20-90	12			
Si (silicon)	12-26	92			
Co (cobalt)	0.1-0.3	<0.13			
B (boron)	0-3.5	2.3			
Sr (strontium)	0.5-10	4.65			
Ba (barium)	0.4-6	1.17			
V (vanadium)	0.1-0.3	<0.07			
Ni (nickel)	0.2-1	0.3			
Ge (germanium)	0.2-0.4	<0.33			
Li (lithium)	0.02-0.45	0.15			
Ag (silver)	0.1-0.6	<0.07			

TOXIC MINERAL	REFERENCE RANGE	TEST VALUE	LOW	TOXIC	VERY TOXIC
Cd (cadmium)	0-0.6	0.33			
Pb (lead)	0-3.5	5.7			
Al (aluminium)	0-5	11.5			
Hg (mercury)	0-2.5	0.30			
As (arsenic)	0-3	0.14			
Be (beryllium)	0-0.25	0.03			
Au (gold)	0-0.5	<0.33			
Pt (platinum)	0-0.5	<0.33			

MINERAL RATIO	REFERENCE RANGE	TEST VALUE
Ca/I	2-10	6.1
Ca/K	5-75	77.4
Cn/Mg	2-60	18.8
Ca/Na	3-50	64.3
Na/K	1-4	1.2
Na/Mg	0.2-4	0.3
Fe/Cu	0.5-3	0.7
Zn/Cu	2-20	14.3

Algal preparations. Burgerstein multi-mineral tablets were given as broad-spectrum multi-mineral agent. Evening primrose oil, fish oil (both Burgerstein) and, sometimes, Mapurit (1 twice daily) Sanum were also given.

(Schüssler salts potassium iodate and magnesium phosphate very often prove helpful in these circumstances. Four daily, sucked like candy.)

The "catalysts of the citric acid cycle" have also proven themselves very much for improving cellular uptake of the trace elements (Heel, ampule set). Drip the contents of an ampule, a drop at a time, once every other day into the nostrils.

Hair Mineral Analysis yielded the following information for this patient

- Diffuse stomach picture
- Problem is located in the intestines
- Immune system is involved, therefore hypoallergenic diet (Dr. Werthmann) necessary
- Cellular uptake problem, therefore catalysts useful
- Toxic, neurotropic stress, treat with diffusion reduction in intestines,
  and antagonists
- Summary: intestinal and milieu treatment top-priority necessity; additionally, dietary allergy

Treatment in this manner brought about a marked improvement within 2 months.

What Information can Hair Mineral Analysis yield?

- Cellular trace element content?
- Toxic metal content? Detoxification necessary?
- Indications of cellular hyperacidity?
- Enteral/cellular resorption?
- Enteral diffusion? (Leaky gut syndrome)
- Main focus of therapy: Mineral salts therapy? Detoxification? Acid-base? Intestinal cleansing?

SUPPLEMENT TO ARTICLE ON HAIR MINERAL ANALYSIS

The above, made multiple references to the importance of an intact intestinal mucous membrane and the intestinal mucous membrane.

The intestinal mucous membrane, by far the largest human organ (approximately 3,230 sq. ft.), is both an uptake and a detoxification organ - and, above all, an immune-system component, in that about 80% of human lymph cells are contained in the Peyer's plaques lining the small intestine mucous membrane. As mentioned above, the intactness of the small intestine (but also the large intestine) mucous membrane is of paramount importance for orthomolecular medicine as well.

The intestinal mucous membrane, in turn, is intimately bound up with the bacterial flora covering it, which make possible part of the mineral salt uptake, and particularly vitamin processing. These intestinal flora, as well as the intestinal mucous membrane cells, must be built up parallel to any orthomolecular substitution therapy, which can be achieved with isopathic and immunobiological remedies, as well as with cellular agents such as Pleo Reb or the Suis products (Heel) derived from swine organs.

The intestinal buildup (using Sanum remedies) described below thus ideally supplements any orthomolecular therapy, and is also a precondition for treating many chronic diseases, particularly hyperactive syndrome.

BUILDING UP THE INTESTINAL FLORA

Milieu Therapy
- Pleo Alkala
- Multi-mineral tablets or ampules

Intestinal Mucous Membrane Buildup
- Dr. Werthmann's Diet (No cow's milk products, no chicken egg products, no mammalian meats)
- Mucosa comp. ampule (Inject 1 ampule twice daily into M25 point, or drink it)

Intestinal flora
- In cases of acute colitis, diarrhea or post-antibiotic: Pleo Not 5X, 1 tablet 3-6 x daily for 3-7 days

- Begin: Pleo Fort 5X, 1 tablet 3 x daily for 14 days
- Then Pleo Pef 4X capsule or drops, 2 weeks
- Then Pleo Sancom drops, 10 drops 2 x daily or Mucokehl and Nigersan for several months

Immune Stimulation

For chronic infections, colitis, etc.

- Pleo Ut and Pleo Rec capsules, 1 each weekly
- Pleo Reb 4X capsules, 1 capsule 2 x daily

TREATING THE HYPERACTIVE CHILD

Definition of Hyperactive Syndrome

Unfortunately, the diagnosis is very often applied to children who don't match up with the in fact fairly strict criteria of the disease picture, which is why we, first of all, include the definition here:

- Onset of behavioral disturbances, before age 5.

- Combination of overactive nonmodulated behaviour with clear lack of attention and a lack of perseverance in carrying out tasks.

- Independent of situation and behavioural disturbances stable over time.

- Combined with disturbance in social behavior.

- Learning disorders can also be present, but not necessarily so. Intelligence disorders are not usually present. Treating the hyperactive child is the domain of regulative medicine and can intervene at the causal level, in that the causes are mostly inner "milieu shifts" and thus "inner disturbed states"; increased histamine formation or trace-element deficiencies, heavy metal burdens and/or vitamin deficiencies lower the nerve cells' or the vegetative ganglia's stimulus threshold.

The hyperactive syndrome is thus mostly a purely organic ailment. It is important to let the little patient and its parents know this, since it is often "psychologized". However, the treatment has to encompass the entire family, particularly where it concerns regulating the daily routine, avoiding toxins and electromagnetic pollution (television) – and of course nutrition.

Treating the hyperactive child must be long-lasting and multifactorial, and adhered to very consistently.

Intestinal Cleansing
Dr. Werthmann's and Dr. Rau's dietary readjustment:

Toxic Metals and their Antagonists

ALUMINIUM:	Calcium, magnesium, vitamin B6, vitamin C
LEAD:	Selenium, calcium, zinc, chromium, methionine, vitamin C
CADMIUM:	Zinc, selenium, methionine, vitamin C, vitamin B6
MERCURY:	Selenium, zinc, methionine, cystine, vitamin C, vitamin E, pectin.

- No milk products, no pork or ham, no anchovies or sardines.
- No canned foods or preserved products.
- No sugar, in particular absolutely no sweet soft drinks such as Coca-Cola, etc.
- No citrus fruits.
- Intestinal flora buildup as per Dr. Rau's plan (see above)

General Remarks Regarding Nutrition
Besides Dr. Werthmann's and Dr. Rau's aforementioned dietary readjustment, the following points must be kept in mind:
- Divide the diet into 5 mealtimes.
- Only organic foods, no preserved foods.
- No sugar or foods containing sugar, no sweet drinks.
- Eat together in a calm, relaxed atmosphere, enjoying the food and allowing enough time.
- No microwave ovens, no overcooking.

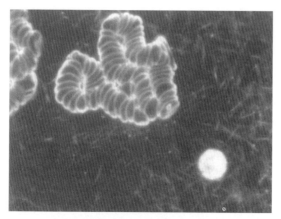

Figures
Darkfield slide of a hyperactive syndrome child (ADDS) typical situation of low oxygen uptake: rouleaux (rolls), very high endobiontic load, dense net of filit. Appearance of an old patient, high degree of degeneration.

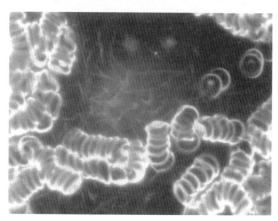

Orthomolecular Therapy
Antagonists: toxic burdens are unusually common among hyperactive children. Every toxic metal has its own specific antagonists.

Orthomolecular Therapy for hyperactive Syndrome
- Evening primrose oil (EPO Burgerstein or Biofrid: 1-2 capsules 3 x daily.
- Fish oil (EPA Burgerstein capsules) alternating with evening primrose oil.
- Multi-mineral tablets (e.g. Burgerstein) 1-2 daily.

- Individually in accordance with the above-named antagonists and results of the Hair Mineral Analysis
- Vitamin E 200 mg daily, possibly with Mg (Mapurit 1 daily, Sanum).
- Vit. B complex (Burgerstein, 1-2 daily).

Isopathic and Immunobiological Therapy for Hyperactive Syndrome

- Must always be combined with orthomolecular therapy.
- There is almost always damage to the intestinal mucous membrane and very often an immune-system disorder (dietary allergy, susceptibility to disease).
- Pleo Sancom drops, 8-10 drops twice daily, ideally a drop at a time into the nostrils.
- Pleo Ut and Pleo Rec drops, rub 1-3 drops daily into each elbow bend.
- Pleo Alkala, alkaline diet.

Complex Homeopathic Therapy for Hyperactive Syndrome

- Catalysts of the citric acid cycle (Heel), one ampule nasally every other day, sequence 1-10, then 10-day break, then start over again.
- On every other intervening day, alternate 1 ampule Cerebrum comp. (Heel) or 1 ampule Coenzyme comp. (Heel).
- Magnesium phosphate 6X or 12X as Schüssler salts.

Dr. Thomas Rau, M.D.
Paracelsus Klinik Lustmühle,
9062 Lustmühle (bei St.Gallen)
Switzerland

Published in Explore! Volume 8 Number 4 1998

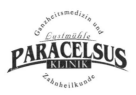

Paracelsus Klinik Lustmühle

Centre for Integrated Biological Medicine and Dentistry
– combining the most advanced diagnostic techniques
with a wide range of natural healing methods for the
rebalancing of the internal milieu and restoration of the
regulatory capacity fundamental to health.

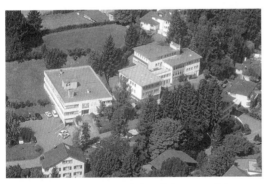

The Paracelsus Klinik Lustmühle, established since 1958, is widely recognised as a centre of excellence for natural medicine. It has now grown into a dynamic team of eighty highly committed people. This includes eight doctors, five dentists, natural health practitioners, nurses and other staff. Absolutely unique to the Paracelsus Klinik is the integration of a holistic dental practice. The clinic has educational facilities for in-house staff training and offers seminars for other practitioners. It also has its own pharmacy for natural remedies and an organic whole food restaurant. The Paracelsus doctors and staff all speak English.

The Paracelsus Klinik specialises in the treatment of chronic and degenerative diseases. The advanced diagnostic tests include dark-field microscopy, biological terrain assessment, electro-acupuncture (Voll), thermography, dental panoramic x-rays, heavy metal evaluation, heart rate variability testing, hair mineral analysis and many others.

Treatments are individualised and are comprised of isopathy according to Enderlein, dietary therapy, acid-alkaline balancing, anthroposophic medicine, homeopathy, neural therapy, osteopathy, oxygenating and ozone therapies, Chinese medicine, herbal remedies, colonics, bioresonance therapy, local and systemic hyperthermia, bodywork, psychospiritual and energetic healing amongst others. The Paracelsus doctors are leading experts on Enderlein therapy, darkfield microscopy and the detoxification of heavy metals. The main clinic is the Paracelsus Klinik Lustmühle, St. Gallen, which is located in the beautiful Swiss mountains, an hour east of Zurich. This clinic provides care on an outpatient basis with nearby hotels enabling people to stay for several weeks at a time. The Paracelsus Klinik Lustmühle treats patients from all over the world. The demand for the Paracelsus model of Integrated Biological Medicine is increasing worldwide and the new Clinica di Cure Biologische Paracelsus Al Ronc is now fulfilling the growing demand for a residential clinic.

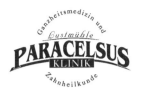

Which Diagnoses are Good to Send to Paracelsus?

AUTOIMMUNE DISEASES
- **Ulcerative Colitis**
- Crohn's Disease
- Lupus Erythematodes

- **Myasthenia Gravis**
- Hashimoto Thyroid disease

- **Rheumatoid Arthritis**

ALL DENTAL AND TOXICO-LOGICAL PROBLEMS
- Heavy Metal Load
- Dental Disturbances

NEUROLOGICAL DISEASES
- Trigeminal Neuralgia

- Multiple Sclerosis
  (not yet in wheel chair or only recently, stopping or healing in 80%)

- Motoneuron Disease
  (Early cases, healing not possible)

"UNCLEAR" DISEASES
- Chronic Fatigue Syndrome
- Multiple Chemical Sensitivity
- Multi Allergies
- Fibromyalgia

CHRONIC INFECTIONS DISEASES
- Hepatitis
- Chronic Sinusitis
- Susceptibility to Infections

CHRONIC INFLAMMATORY OR INFECTIOUS DISEASES
- Eosinophilic Pneumonia
- Chronic lung fibrosis/Asthma

- Chronic Osteomyelitis
- Chronic glomerulonephritis
  (no dialysis patients!)
- Chronic Prostatitis
- All Lumbovertebral Diseases
  (also Disc Herniations)

CANCER AND TUMOROUS DISEASES

- Prostate Cancer (all stages)
- Breast Cancer (early stages and after Chemoth.)
- All other Cancers, but please evaluate individually with Dr. Rau

Dr. Thomas Rau, M.D.
Paracelsus Klinik Lustmühle,
9062 Lustmühle (bei St.Gallen)
Switzerland

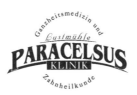

Clinica Paracelsus Al Ronc

The new Biological Medicine clinic in Switzerland for intensive isopathic therapy: a daughter clinic of Paracelsus Lustmühle

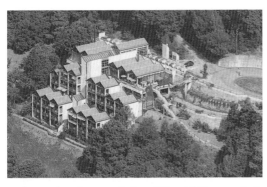

In September 2001 the first and to date only clinic practising Integrated Biological Medicine was opened in Castaneda in Canton Ticino. Therapies according to Prof. Enderlein are practised in combination with intensive milieu therapy and orthomolecular medicine. The Al Ronc clinic uses the same programme of treatments as its "parent clinic", the Paracelsus Klinik Lustmühle, the strengths of which lie in the treatment of "difficult" illnesses which orthodox medicine hardly begins to tackle or about which we still know too little – for example: allergies/asthma, chronic immune diseases, chronic fatigue syndrome (CFS), unclear "vegetative" and toxic clinical pictures (heavy metals), auto-immune diseases and tumours.

Both the clinics advocate "Integrated Biological Medicine" as developed at the Paracelsus Klinik Lustmühle under the direction of Dr Thomas Rau and as practised and taught for many years. Integrated Biological Medicine starts from the assumption that a human being is a dynamic system and that therefore illness is not a static condition but a constantly changing process, which is dependent on the person's regulatory capacity. Therefore, for chronic illnesses to be healed, the revitalisation force of the person must be strengthened. To achieve this, Biological Medicine unites traditional and modern methods of natural healing in its treatment plan – for example: isopathy, milieu therapy, orthomolecular medicine, medicine which concentrates on the focus of a disorder, neural therapy, homeopathy and homotoxicology – and combines them individually according to the patient's constitution.

The Paracelsus Clinic Al Ronc is a clinic for intensive in-patient treatment. It is designed to accommodate patients with the disorders described above, as well as patients with nebulous diseases such as psycho-vegetative exhaustion, chronic vague gastro-intestinal problems, chronic viral diseases (herpes, hepatitis C, etc), cancer patients in intervals between courses of other types of treatments and people who need generally building up but do not simply want to passively submit to orthodox medical treatment.

In the clinic, courses of Biological medical treatment are carried out actively, with a specific aim and tailored to the individual; these may be based on a special diet or fasting or be designed with the aim of building up the patient. A team of motivated doctors and therapists, all enthusiasts for this type of treatment, combine several types of natural therapy with deep-acting Sanum therapy and immune-biological therapy in order to retune and restore the patient's inner milieu, including the health-promoting Paracelsus Diet (low in animal protein, alkaline, low in allergens and builds up the flora and activity of the intestine).

The Paracelsus Clinic Al Ronc specialises in intensive therapies designed to support detoxification, excretion, cleansing of the bowel and the building up of weakened organs. The following complete courses of treatment are offered as a particular speciality for complaints for which up to now treatment has hardly been satisfactory:

- Paracelsus treatment to build up the bowel (dysbiosis, colitis, immune disorders)

- Paracelsus heavy metal detoxification (neurological disorders)

- Intensive Paracelsus strengthening treatment to regenerate and remove blockages, e.g. in cases of hypertonia, cardiac diseases, build-up of morbid matter

- Paracelsus joint and rheumatism treatment with deep de-acidification and strengthening of the joints, for rheumatism, arthritis, non-articular rheumatism syndrome, etc.

The Paracelsus Clinic Al Ronc is there to help independent, thinking, active people who do not simply want to take a passive "recuperative break" but wish to take an active role in influencing their health intensively. A course of treatment is the beginning of a new orientation that permanently re-tunes and strengthens the person's inner milieu and their ability to regenerate. Patients receive comprehensive Biological treatment and are given guidance as to what they themselves can do in terms of diet and a healthy lifestyle. The treatment is thus a practice-oriented, intensive period of teaching to benefit the patient's future.

Contact address:
Clinica Paracelsus Al Ronc
CH-6540 Castenada, Switzerland

Tel. +41 (0)91 820 40 40
Fax +41 (0)91 820 40 41
info@alronc.ch
www.alronc.ch

MYRO FLEX THERAPIE

- PSA TEST RESULTS
- TPS TEST RESULTS
- THYROID NEURAL THERAPY
- EDTA CHELATION